REACH

9 HABITS TO GET IN SHAPE,

YOUR

CONTROL STRESS AND

PEAK

PERFORM AT YOUR BEST

ALEX PEDLEY

R^ethink

First published in Great Britain in 2021 by Rethink Press (www.rethinkpress.com)

For my soulmate, Brooke. Without your support, patience and encouragement, this book would never have been finished. And for my two children, Harry and Lila, who inspire me daily.

Contents

Introduction

Some people seem to live a healthy lifestyle with ease. They're often called 'fitness fanatics' or 'health nuts'. They make the right choices when it comes to food; they enjoy working out; they're in good shape. Meanwhile, they work in challenging jobs, run busy social lives and have time for their families.

These people appear to have hit the sweet spot – they've found the balance between being busy and having fun and living well. They'll happily talk about their journey with you and try to persuade you to do the same thing. That's because they live with their ideal weight, expect to wake up feeling energised, move without aches and pains, and have confidence in their bodies.

They don't have extra determination – they've chosen a lifestyle. They've taken an approach to health and well-being that's different from that of many people.

Some people yo-yo from one diet to another while intermittently taking part in workout classes they don't particularly enjoy. Others exercise regularly but never seem to achieve the results that their efforts deserve. Then there are the people who gave up trying ages ago, or never started in the first place.

The fact that you're reading this tells me that you'd like to be in the first group. Who wouldn't? But I'm not here to tell you that there's a secret formula or a quick-fix solution. Unfortunately, it simply doesn't work that way – and if anyone tries to sell you a system that does, turn around and walk away.

Although there is no secret, there is a set of scientifically proven principles that, if followed, will enable you to achieve your ideal body weight, better manage stress and get into great shape.

You won't need to do high-intensity workouts or go on a restrictive diet, but you will need to put in effort and change your thinking. Before we dig into that, though, let me introduce myself.

I began my career nearly twenty years ago working as a coach within large corporate companies based all over the City of London. These were the boom times, where bankers and brokers worked hard and played harder.

As a young man from East London, I loved the environment – highly paid and influential people rushing around engrossed in business conversations or making their way to the next meeting or back to the trading floor.

I also loved the party lifestyle that followed a busy day at the office. I made friends with many of the people who used the fitness centres and joined them in their after-work festivities, which often involved partying late into the night. Times were good.

Then, in 2008, the banking crisis hit and the business world changed dramatically. At the time, I was travelling the world, but when I returned in 2009, I found the environment very different. It had moved away from the excesses enjoyed pre-crash. Things were more controlled. Yet, the insane working hours and high levels of stress remained.

Instead of looking at the stressful lives that the employees were living and thinking that this wasn't the kind of life I wanted, I went in the opposite direction. Coaching and socialising with wealthy bankers, lawyers and managing directors had opened me up to the lifestyle they lived and made me want the same.

I applied the work ethic of these highly successful people to my own life. I trained clients back-to-back for much of the day with minimal breaks. This allowed me to build common ground with my clients – when they came down to see me for coaching after all-day meetings, I knew how they felt and how draining the lifestyle could be.

The large number of clients that I coached week on week, year on year, gave me a unique perspective into how a corporate business is run and the health and well-being challenges that come with it. I coached and became friends with CEOs, directors, analysts, personal assistants, even their chefs and chauffeurs. I heard stories of how each level within a large blue-chip company comes with its unique issues.

Working so closely with employees from all levels within a massive institution allowed me to see how two people from the same team, doing relatively similar work, could have quite different experiences. A situation that would allow one person to thrive might break another.

The difference was strikingly obvious; the people who thrived in this world had found balance. They worked just as hard as their colleagues but also had structure. They were driven by routines. They found pockets of time to exercise, eat a well-rounded diet and recover. This allowed them to stay mentally sharp and in good physical shape.

As my knowledge increased – both through working closely with these people and through consuming books about fitness, nutrition, sleep, stress management and behavioural change – I applied what I was learning to my life and helped my clients do the same. The results that I saw personally and in the lives of the people I coached were truly transformational. It wasn't one particular type of workout or diet; it was several core lifestyle choices, implemented progressively, that made the real impact.

It also became clear to me how ineffective short-term solutions are when it comes to getting fit. Unfortunately, the fitness industry does little to change this perception. High-intensity workouts are still billed as the best solution to get in shape, and a new type of restrictive diet seems to be on offer daily. This approach is broken. It's time to follow a different strategy.

If you deal with stressful situations regularly, spend much of the day seated, eat on the go, don't feel as if you have enough time in the day and often wake up tired, then taking part in intense workouts and dieting isn't the solution. Don't waste your valuable time and energy.

I've written this book to show you that there's a better way, an easier way, a more sustainable way to achieve your ideal body, manage stress and reach peak condition. I'll introduce you to simple steps that will allow you to transform how you look and feel. The results will last a lifetime.

This approach isn't easy; no lifestyle change is. But it is easier and more sustainable than many common approaches. In Part One, I'll outline why the current approach isn't working for the masses and the importance of habits in a busy lifestyle.

In Part Two, we'll explore the nine lifestyle habits in three core areas – exercise, nutrition and recovery – that will transform how you look, feel and perform.

First, you'll learn how to build a strong base that will allow you to move with more freedom and become the best athletic version of yourself.

Next, you'll learn a simple three-step way to make healthy food choices – structure, energy balance, 80/20 – so that you're adequately fuelling your body for peak performance and can achieve your ideal body weight.

Finally, you'll learn powerful ways to start your day off right, better manage stress and create a bedtime routine that ensures you get good-quality sleep consistently.

In Part Three, I'll introduce a system to help you make the best possible start on your transformational journey, pinpoint what you want to achieve and identify the deeper reason you wish to make a change.

Each chapter can be read on its own, and you're welcome to search out the information you're most interested in learning, but to get the most from this book, I advise you to read it in order.

Many things look good on paper but don't work well in reality, so I've made sure nothing in this book is unachievable or unrealistic – quite the opposite. The systems are user-friendly and will work within your busy schedule. You can blend a successful career, family life and social life while maintaining good health and well-being.

If you're reading this book, you're ready to achieve genuine, long-lasting change when it comes to how you look, feel and perform. The strategies in this book will give you all you need to reach peak condition. Get ready to begin a transformational journey that will last a lifetime.

PART ONE

IT'S TIME TO CHANGE THE APPROACH

1
Habits

In my home office one afternoon, I spoke with my friend via a video call about how much he was struggling with work. He explained that the unrelenting work hours and the sheer volume of work that he needed to complete after all-day meetings meant he found it challenging to find time for himself.

The situation had become worse since he began working from home. He'd fallen entirely out of the routine he'd been in while working in the office, and this meant he struggled to find the time to work out and even go for a walk – previously essential parts of his day.

He explained that his eating habits had also changed. Before, his personal assistant would grab his lunch.

Now, he had to prepare it himself, which meant he'd eat whatever was available in his fridge. This often led to poor choices.

In the evening, he had trouble switching off. This affected both the quality and quantity of his sleep. He'd also gained weight and felt out of shape. He wasn't in a good way.

I asked my friend about his routine – in particular, how he started and ended the day. He explained that first thing in the morning was one of the only times he didn't have meetings. It was also when the house was quiet because his two young children were still asleep. He'd begin working almost straight away, checking his phone for emails and getting on with his current project.

He'd often check emails up until the last half hour before going to bed, which meant that when it was time to sleep, he struggled to switch off and would lie there playing the day's events in his mind. He'd finally fall asleep exhausted. Then, around 3am, he'd wake up with his mind racing and would struggle to fall asleep again.

He often woke up in the morning feeling tired. He'd drink a strong coffee before repeating it all the next day. He said he felt as if he were on a hamster wheel and couldn't get off.

My friend's story isn't unique. I hear similar stories all the time. Many people struggle to balance looking after number one with a career and family life. If work becomes hectic or an unexpected change happens in their life, they slip into a bad routine. Before long, their lifestyle changes become ingrained habits.

You may feel as if you have no time to exercise, eat well or switch off. You may wake up in the middle of the night with your mind racing, feel tired in the morning and have no energy for the day.

It doesn't have to be this way. You have everything you need to turn your life around. I'm going to teach you simple but highly effective strategies to create time in your day for yourself, so that you can concentrate on the things that matter most to you.

Many of the things you'll learn in this book might seem counterintuitive. You'll need to let go of some old ideas about exercise, nutrition and recovery and embrace new ones.

If you're ready to do that, then read on.

The 5Ss

Time stress is one of the primary causes of falling into unhealthy habits. All-day meetings, early starts and late nights at the office, impending project deadlines and family commitments are causes of time stress.

It may begin in situations such as starting a new job role or welcoming a new child. To adapt to the extra time demands you start to grab food whenever possible, stop exercising for a few weeks, go to bed later or give yourself less opportunities for time to yourself. Although at the start none of these examples cause too many issues, but over time, these small changes in your lifestyle begin to compound, leaving you feeling more tired, stressed and out of shape.

What was once a quick fix to address a busy period has now become an ingrained habit. These lifestyle choices often lead to what I call the 5Ss of busy professionals. These are five common problems I've witnessed time and again in my career coaching high performers. Most will have at least three if not more of them.

Without a clear strategy to adapt to a lifestyle that involves eating on the run, spending long periods seated and working long hours, the 5Ss are inevitable.

The good news is that you can improve each of them with the right approach. Let's look at each one.

Soft body

A soft body is one carrying excess body fat. A certain level of body fat is normal and healthy; what I'm referring to is having more body fat than you feel comfortable with. Most people know when they're holding more body fat than is healthy for their size and shape.

It's caused by periods of overeating and a lack of exercise, both common for people who are busy and work in sedentary jobs.

Out of *shape*

The nature of modern life means that there is less reason to stay active. If we don't exercise, we become out of shape. It's as simple as that.

As a result, we can feel out of breath after running for a bus or struggle to lift something we once could.

Stiff joints

Spending long periods in the same position can cause stiff joints. This could manifest as lower back pain when you bend to pick something up from the floor, sore knees when walking downstairs or shoulder pain when reaching for something.

Although there can be many causes for these ailments, joint immobility is a primary one.

Stressed out

Many people move from one busy situation to the next, never allowing themselves any down time. They feel rushed, which can cause anxiety and a sense that there's not enough time in the day.

Not all stress is bad. It's a matter of how much time you spend in a stressed-out state.

Sleepless nights

Late nights at the office or working from home, early starts and young children are common reasons for not getting enough sleep.

Many people struggle to switch off after a busy day, so they're either unable to fall asleep or they wake up in the middle of the night with an overactive mind (or both).

Each of the 5Ss can impact the other. For example, being stressed out at work can affect sleep. If you don't sleep well, your body boosts its levels of stress hormones. The following day, you'll feel more stressed out. You'll then find it harder to fall asleep when night comes – and on it goes. Poor sleep quality will also impact your ability to recover from a workout and can cause sugar cravings.

This is just one example of how the 5Ss are intertwined. It's important to focus on improving each area to get the best from your body.

You may identify with one or more of the 5Ss. Most people do. Focusing on improving the 5Ss and implementing a wellness strategy is crucial to your health, happiness and performance. This doesn't require a complete overhaul of your routine; in fact, I would strongly advise against taking that approach.

Just as each of the 5Ss builds up over time as the result of poor lifestyle choices, reversing the effects of the 5Ss requires you to progressively introduce healthier lifestyle choices and build new habits.

EXERCISE

Do you suffer from any of the 5Ss?

If so, think about how your lifestyle habits might be impacting each area.

As you read through this book, make notes on the strategies discussed to undo the effects of the 5Ss and begin implementing them into your routine.

Forming habits

As unbelievable as it might sound, you make most of your daily decisions on autopilot. Studies show that 40% of our daily activities are habitual.[1]

In his book *Thinking, Fast and Slow*, Nobel Prize–winning psychologist Daniel Kahneman suggests that we have two modes of decision making, which he coined System One and System Two.

System One is defined as being unconscious and fast and requiring minimal effort. It is automatic and based on previous experiences and memory. We have no control over it; it is involuntary. System Two, on the other hand, is deliberate and slow and requires more mental effort.[2]

When the day is in full flow, we often revert to System One to make decisions. If we had to rely on high-level thinking, we would quickly become overwhelmed by the constant flood of information.

We can relate this to health and well-being decisions. When we're busy, we'll revert to what we've done before because it takes less mental energy to do so.

Although the term 'habit' often carries negative connotations, you wouldn't be able to survive without your habits. From tying the same shoe first to starting on the same section of teeth when brushing, you habitually begin certain actions in the same way. You do this without even thinking. If you didn't have unconscious habits, you wouldn't be able to function. If you live with a partner, when you go to bed this evening, try getting into their side of the bed and see what they say; I bet you that they won't be happy. You'll be disrupting their routine.

All habits start with a conscious decision – they then become unconscious behaviours.

Perhaps you enjoy a glass of red wine one evening after work. It helps you relax, so you decide to do the same the following night. Then the action is repeated until, before you know it, you've created a habit of having a glass of wine each evening. It doesn't seem to be a problem, as it doesn't directly affect your ability to function the next day, but you understand that you should probably cut down.

You decide to stop for a few weeks, but then, after a difficult day, you have a glass of wine. This continues for a few nights. Soon, you've fallen back into the habit of drinking every night.

This is just one example of a habit that can easily slip into your routine but can be hard to remove.

In his book *The Power of Habit,* Charles Duhigg discusses a 'simple neurological loop at the core of every habit, a loop that consists of three parts: a cue, a routine and a reward'.[3]

When we repeat a conscious action consistently enough, we create an association between the routine and the cue. Let's continue using the wine example. The cue may be getting home from work, the routine is pouring a glass and drinking it, and the reward is the relaxed feeling the alcohol gives you.

Initially the thought arises in the prefrontal cortex, which is in a part of the brain called the frontal lobe.

When repeated enough times, the action becomes automatic and moves to the basal ganglia. At this point, we are often unaware of the habit, generally only thinking about it if it has a detrimental effect on us.

Whether they're good or bad, all habits are formed when a behaviour is consciously repeated. This includes wellness habits. How you eat, how you exercise, how you approach sleep, how you manage stress – all these habits will compound and will ultimately impact your physique, your performance, your health and your happiness.

If you're successful in your career, it's because of your work habits. If you have financial freedom, it's because of your money habits. If you want to get in great shape, you must have good wellness habits.

This is where your focus must lie – create the right habits to accelerate your transformation journey.

As we've discussed, creating a new habit requires taking conscious and consistent actions. Your efforts will soon compound and you'll build momentum, creating a snowball effect. Over time, the habit will become ingrained into your life, and you'll identify with the new lifestyle choice.

We're going to explore systems and strategies to undo many of the impacts of twenty-first-century living, so that you can live a healthier and more fulfilled life. First, though, we'll look at the most common approaches to getting in shape and the pitfalls that come with following these strategies.

Key points

- We do 40% of our daily actions without really thinking. All habits follow a similar pattern, starting with a trigger, followed by an action and finishing with a reward. Whatever you do consistently will eventually become an ingrained habit.

- During stressful and busy periods, it is easy to slip into unhealthy lifestyle choices. Over time, these choices can lead to what I call the 5Ss of busy professionals: soft body, out of shape, stiff joints, stressed out and sleepless nights.

- You don't need a complete overhaul to counter the 5Ss. Instead, focus on progressively introducing healthier lifestyle choices and building new habits.

2
There Is No Quick Fix

As we sat down in a busy coffee shop overlooking London Bridge during the mid-morning rush of people getting their caffeine fix, my former client and good friend looked at someone who was tucking into a chocolate croissant. She then gave me a wry smile and said, 'That was my breakfast of choice before I met you.'

I laughed before asking how she was. She updated me on her life before the conversation drifted towards her friend, Jane, who'd just completed a twelve-week transformation programme.

Jane, a thirty-nine-year-old digital analyst, worked from home most days. She was fond of an evening glass of wine and spent most of her day sitting in her home office in front of her computer.

For most of her life, she had yo-yoed between exercising and not exercising, and between going on a diet and giving up a diet. Her weight also yo-yoed.

After going the longest period in her adult life without exercising and generally eating unhealthily, she was more overweight than she'd ever been and felt, in her words, 'embarrassingly out of shape'.

She'd found a transformation programme that promised fast results – so she'd signed up.

The programme involved four intense workouts each week. Meanwhile, she restricted her calorie intake to no more than 1,300 per day. The programme pushed her to her limit, but she managed to keep at it because she'd paid for it. Plus, it lasted only twelve weeks, so she hung on in the hope that she'd see the reward for her effort.

She did see positive results – she lost weight and felt fitter. It was when the programme ended that the problems arose. She found herself burnt out from the experience and longing, physically and mentally, for food. The old habits began to creep back in.

She'd maintained a lower calorie intake while on the programme but hadn't learned proper eating habits, so she found it difficult to sustain. The workouts were so intense that she had little chance of continuing to do them in the long term.

When she returned to her old habits, she regained the lost weight, and then gained even more. She felt stressed out and back where she'd started.

Essentially, she'd done a hypothetical sprint when she needed to go on a steady jog. This is where so many people go wrong.

The temptation to change everything can be strong – lay everything on the line and hang in there until the results start showing. It seems to make sense that the harder you work and the more restrictive the diet, the quicker you'll see results.

But it simply doesn't work like that.

High-intensity workouts and restrictive diets will only increase the likelihood of mental and physical over-whelm – thereby increasing the chances of returning to old habits.

Exercise and healthy eating are the solution. It's how you approach these that determines how sustainable the results will be. Making small, consistent changes is the key to a lifelong transformation. Build the right foundations and you will be able to adapt to busy periods and life's challenges.

However, making small and consistent changes is the opposite of how some people approach trying to get in shape. They bypass building the necessary foundations and head straight for more severe measures. In this chapter, we look at why restrictive diets and intense workouts are not a sustainable approach to losing weight for most people.

Exercise alone isn't an effective weight-loss strategy

As I waited on my bike, I watched people filter into the class I was about to teach. The class was scheduled to begin at 1.20pm and, as always, most of the participants rushed into the studio at around 1.15pm and saved their preferred bike by placing their towel on it before heading to the changing rooms to get into their workout gear. Half the people who came in were busy checking their phones and sending emails up to the last minute before the class commenced. Many of the attendees had finished a meeting just before the class.

After a 5-minute warm-up, we moved into a high-intensity interval session. I knew everyone wanted to work hard, so I pushed them. The class was a mix of short sprints followed by an active recovery – jumps (moving between a standing and seated position on the bike) and longer intervals. The studio mirrors clouded over with condensation as the temperature in the room rose from the body heat.

Near the end of the 45-minute class, a number of the participants shifted back into work mode. Some left a few minutes early to beat the rush for the showers, so they'd have just enough time to pick up some lunch, still sweating from the workout, and make their way to their next challenging meeting. Only a few had enough time for a quick chat and a stretch at the end of the session.

At the start of my career, I regularly took high-intensity classes and endorsed an intense training style both in my own workouts and when coaching clients. I pushed as hard as possible in each session, knowing that people often associated good coaches with those who did so. This mentality can lead to a situation where the client expects an intense workout because they believe it's the best way to get in shape. The coach takes them through a hard session as this is what the client wants, and the client leaves the session feeling wiped out but thinks this is a good thing.

This has led to a culture where people believe that the only way to get in shape is to work out intensely. If they are not pouring with sweat and crawling out of a session, they haven't worked hard enough, and the workout wasn't effective.

High-intensity interval training has become synonymous with burning calories, so many people believe that the harder the workout, the greater the energy expenditure.

You'll burn more calories doing intense anaerobic activities than you will when performing aerobic exercise. Consider, however, that working out makes up roughly 10% of your total daily energy expenditure (TDEE) – the small number of extra calories burned from a high-intensity workout is not quite enough to make your exercise selection based on it.

In 2017, Harvard Health Publishing released data on the number of calories burned by people of varying body weights within a 30-minute workout. One of the results showed that during a moderate-intensity bike ride session, a person of 57 kg (125 lb) burned only 210 calories. Another result showed that in circuit training, a higher-intensity activity, a 57-kg person burned just 240 calories.[4]

To put it into perspective, a standard 51-gram Mars bar contains 229 calories.

One of the benefits of high-intensity workouts often discussed is that they increase excess post-exercise oxygen consumption (EPOC). EPOC is the amount of oxygen needed to restore homeostasis – the body's stable internal environment.[5] Think about the time it takes for the engine of your car to cool down after a long journey, this is similar to how the body recovers from a workout. This means your body can continue to burn a high number of calories for up to 48 hours after you've finished your workout, although the number of calories burned and the duration it lasts may be overstated.

Research has shown that the intensity needed to stimulate a prolonged period of EPOC would not be tolerated by most non-athletes. Unless you are already in great shape, you will struggle to work hard enough for long enough to maintain an elevated metabolism. You may burn slightly more calories post workout but far fewer than many who promote an intense form of exercise within the fitness community would have you believe.[6]

Exercise is a means to improve your body's performance. It will make you stronger, fitter and more mobile, and it plays an important role in weight management. It's not an effective weight-loss strategy when used in isolation.

If weight loss is your primary goal, finding the right balance between the calories you consume and the calories you expend is where you want to place most of your attention. In the same way that there is a misconception about the number of calories we can expend from intense exercise, there is also a belief that restrictive dieting is the best solution for weight loss. As you will see, it is not necessarily true.

Restrictive dieting rarely leads to sustained weight loss

While in a restaurant with my partner one day, I noticed four women in their mid-thirties ordering food. Three, who were petite, selected a starter and a main, but the fourth, who would be classed as overweight for her height, asked for only a starter. When the waiter asked if she was sure that the starter was all she wanted, she said that she wasn't hungry.

When the starters came out, the women commented on how much they enjoyed them and chatted happily. Then the main courses arrived. The woman who hadn't ordered one watched her friends eating and looked slightly uncomfortable. She ate some bread as her friends enjoyed and discussed their meals.

This situation isn't uncommon. People often say that they're not hungry or that they're on a diet when social-ising. If the person is trying to lose weight, they avoid eating around others. Although it's not out of the ordi-nary, it can lead to a destructive relationship with food.

It's now more common to talk about food to be avoided instead of food to be enjoyed. This has led to a society where many people consume food and then feel guilty after, promising themselves and others that they'll return to their 'diet' the next day.

In 2016, a survey by Mintel showed that 48% of Brits had tried to lose weight that year, with 64% of those saying they dieted 'all or most of the time'.[7]

Dieting is now a multibillion-pound industry. There are so many on the market, it's easy to become confused about which approach to take. Although the diets all proclaim to offer the secret formula for weight loss, obesity numbers continue to rise.[8] The 2019 Health Survey for England estimated that 28% of adults in England were obese and 36.2% were overweight – that's one-third of the population.[9]

In a review of thirty-one published studies on long-term weight loss, a team of researchers at UCLA found that over two to five years, although people initially lost between 5% and 10% of their body weight, most regained all the weight lost. Tracy Mann, the lead researcher, said that the results were conclusive: 'Diets do not lead to sustained weight loss or health benefits for the majority of people.'[10]

Many diets prescribe drastically restricting calorie intake. Again, this approach works, but only for a short period.

EXERCISE

Consider the following questions:

- Have you ever tried a weight-loss diet?
- If yes, how did it work for you?
- Were you able to maintain it?
- How did it make you feel?

The Minnesota Starvation Experiment

One of the most famous studies on extreme calorie restriction took place during the Second World War. In 1950, the results of the Minnesota Starvation Experiment were published in *The Biology of Human Starvation*.[11] The initial purpose of the study was to determine what would happen if rationing continued after the war and turned into starvation.

Thirty-six men were part of the year-long study, in which they were required to lose 25% of their average body weight. Their diet contained foods that were high in carbohydrates and low in protein, including potatoes, root vegetables and bread, a typical diet in Europe at the time.

The experiment was split into four stages.

Stage one (twelve weeks) was the control phase. This was to determine how many calories each of the men needed per day to maintain their weight.

Stage two (twenty-four weeks) was the semi-starvation phase. Each man was restricted to 1,570 calories per day.

Stage three (twelve weeks) was the restricted rehabilitation stage. At this point, the number of calories, vitamins and proteins required to bring the men back to a healthy weight was determined.

Stage four (eight weeks) was the unrestricted rehabilitation stage. Twelve of the men were persuaded to stay
after the trial to assess what happened when they were
allowed to eat what they wanted but were monitored
for calorie intake.

Each participant was required to walk 22 miles per
week, to expend more calories than they consumed
each day. They also worked 15 hours in the lab per
week and took part in educational activities for 25
hours per week throughout the experiment.

The findings were eye-opening.

In the semi-starvation stage, the men soon showed a
remarkable decline in energy and a 21% reduction in
strength. They became emaciated, their body temperature, heart rate and sex drive declined, and they were
irritable, anxious and withdrawn.

They became obsessed with food, and mealtimes
became the highlight of the day. The men became agi-
tated if the meal was delayed, and they often spent time
discussing and reading about food. Cheating became a
big issue as the participants battled with almost uncon-
trollable urges to find food. As a result, they weren't
allowed outside of the lab's confines without a 'buddy'.

Although the participants grew skeletal thin, they
believed they were fat, and the researchers noted similarities to anorexia.

In the restricted rehabilitation stage, the men were split into four groups. Each group received either an extra 400, 800, 1,200 or 1,600 calories than they had in the semi-starvation phase, so the researchers could figure out which amount best supported the recovery. The participants on an extra 400 calories showed no signs of recovery, even with extra vitamins or protein – their bodies just wanted the calorie deficit to be reversed.

In the final eight weeks, and even though participants had been warned not to do so, several men engaged in extreme overeating when left to their own devices. Some of them feasted on as many as 11,500 calories in a single day.

While each participant's weight declined by about 25%, their percentage of body fat fell by almost 70%, and their muscle mass decreased by about 40%.

During the controlled rehabilitation, a more significant proportion of the weight regained was fat. Eight months into the rehabilitation, the volunteers returned to near their original body weight but with about a 140% increase in body fat.

In the Minnesota Starvation Experiment, the men were in the semi-starvation phase if they consumed fewer than 1,600 calories, which is more than many modern diets allow. This study's results should have changed how we see extreme calorie restriction to this day, but unfortunately, they had little effect. When people want to lose weight, they drastically cut calories and end up longing for food, making it hard for them to stick to the diet.

Just as in the Minnesota Starvation Experiment the participants suffered with hormonal disruption, food cravings, reduction in muscle mass and reduced energy, so too do many dieters. This is why the approach is often unsustainable.

This isn't to say that severe calorie restriction is ineffective. The participants continued to lose weight right to the end of the study, although the rate of weight loss slowed. It's the sustainability of the method that's the problem, not the effectiveness.

If weight loss is your goal, you'll need to consume fewer calories than you expend, but you don't have to choose an extreme option. A smaller calorie deficit will still lead to weight loss, but it will avoid many of the unpleasant side effects of severe calorie restriction and, although challenging, it's much more sustainable and will leave you with energy to exercise.

Exercise and nutrition should improve your performance. They should increase your energy, make you more focused and enable you to gain confidence in your body. High-intensity workouts and extreme calorie restriction often have the opposite effect.

To get in shape and stay that way, your focus needs to be on adapting habits rather than looking for quick fixes. This is how you achieve the kind of transformation that lasts a lifetime.

A gradual approach

The strategy to lose weight and maintain a healthy weight is relatively simple: consume fewer calories than you expend.

There are many things that impact your ability to be able to achieve this goal: the type of food you consume, your sleep quality, stress levels, resistance training and your activity level. We will look at how each of these impacts weight loss and a strategy to improve them in upcoming chapters. Another important factor is the speed of weight loss.

There is often a disparity between expected weight loss and what is recommended and achievable. One study looked at sixty obese women and asked them to rate how much weight they expected to lose over forty-eight weeks. They were asked to choose their ideal, happy, acceptable and disappointing levels of weight loss. At the end of the trial, 47% of the patients had failed even to achieve the amount of weight loss that they had classed as disappointing.[12]

It is completely understandable to expect quick results. If you do not find the right balance between effort and reward, your chances of sustaining the journey will reduce. However, it is important to differentiate between consistent progress and rapid weight loss that is unsustainable. People who lose weight too quickly invariably rebound for many of the reasons documented in the Minnesota Starvation Experiment. The key is to focus on taking an approach which enables you to lose weight and keep it off and setting realistic expectations of what is achievable.

For most people, a weight-loss goal of 0.2–1 kg per week is a good rate. If you lose 0.5 kg every week for the next year on average, you will lose 26 kg, or 4 stone. Half a kilogram per week doesn't sound impressive, but 26 kg is an amazing transformation. By taking this approach, you will build new habits, and this greatly increases the chances of maintaining the reduced weight.

By taking a more gradual approach, you will ensure that you are able to fuel your body adequately to perform in your workouts and daily life. You will also be able to supply your body with adequate nutrients to support your immune system.

Begin by identifying the underlying eating habits that have led to weight gain, create structure so that making healthier choices is easier, find the right energy balance to achieve your aesthetic goal and create a well-rounded diet. We will talk about how to achieve each of these goals in Part Two.

EXERCISE

Think about your current approach to exercise and diet:

- Do you envisage being able to maintain it for the next year and beyond?
- Are you able to build on this approach so that you see consistent improvement?

If the answer to either of those questions is 'no', it may be time to change your approach.

Key points

- Intense workouts do not burn considerably more calories than less intense workouts. Do not make your exercise selection with weight loss as the primary goal.

- Restricted dieting isn't a sustainable weight-loss strategy and often leads to a rebound effect.

- To achieve sustainable weight loss, it is important to focus on consistent progress instead of rapid weight loss. This way you will be able to maintain the results you achieve. This is true for all wellness habits.

3
Your Workout Is Only As Good As Your Recovery

Imagine this scenario. You're on a three-day hiking vacation in America with a friend, exploring beautiful mountain scenery. This trip is meant to be an escape from the stress of day-to-day life.

A few miles into your trek, you spot three large kittens near the trail. Then you see the mother. A cougar. She growls at you.

Fear takes hold of your body, triggering a flood of stress hormones. Your heart pumps more oxygen to your muscles; your lungs dilate and your breathing speeds up.

As the cougar begins to pursue you, you start walking backwards, keeping an eye on her, both thinking about your escape and not wanting to confront the big cat.

More oxygen is sent to your brain, making your senses sharper. More blood, sugar and fat are released into your system, boosting your energy. Your body is now on red alert and ready for action.

The cougar disappears into the woods but soon comes back into view, this time beside you. She appears to be stalking you, ready to pounce. You continue walking backwards. A few minutes later, the angry cat growls, ears pinned back and teeth bared. She springs toward you.

Fortunately, she doesn't attack.

The exhausting encounter has been going on for 5 minutes now, and you think you have enough distance to bend down, grab a rock and throw it at the cougar. Sure enough, you do, and the cougar spins around and runs back down the trail to her cubs. You take a deep breath while muttering a few expletives. You're safe and out of danger. It's now that your body begins to recover.

You've just been through the first stage of the stress response often referred to as 'fight, flight or freeze'. It's an evolutionary response to danger.

Although most people in the Western world rarely find themselves in this kind of situation, many spend a large portion of their day in a state of fight, flight or freeze.

The word '*stress*' is now used regularly in general conversation, but this hasn't always been the case.

Hans Selye first introduced general adaptation syndrome (GAS), now more commonly known as the stress response, in his book *The Stress of Life*. To find out how the stress response worked, Selye experimented on rodents. He applied various stressors, such as poking and prodding and heat and cold, and found that no matter the stressor, there was always a generalised response to it.

Selye discovered that if he removed the stressor quickly enough, the mice would adapt and become better at resisting that stressor. If he left the stressor there too long, the mice would become less resistant to it and, in many cases, would even die. The key was giving them enough of the stressor to adapt, but not too much.[13]

Psychological and psychosocial stressors, such as an impending work deadline or a difficult relationship, stimulate many of the same stress responses as physical stress, such as that generated by a hard workout.

Usually, the stressors are so subtle that they cause little effect straight away, but over time they begin to take their toll. There's only so much stress that we can adapt to at any one time.

Think of your tolerance to stress as a bucket and the stressor as water. During the day, you add water to the bucket at different rates. Your day might look something like this: you leave the house after a disagreement with your partner; you jump on a packed train; you go straight into a pressurised meeting; at lunchtime, you walk to the nearby gym in near-freezing temperatures; you then do a high-intensity workout. Good or bad, each one of these situations is a stressor that adds water to the bucket.

If you don't have recovery strategies in place, you'll get to the point where there's no more room in the bucket, and it will overflow. If the bucket overflows consistently over a long period, it will deteriorate until it can't hold any water any more – this is when burnout occurs.

Stress itself isn't the problem; uncontrolled stress is. To thrive in an intense environment, it is crucial to be able to switch gears and adapt to stressful situations. This is something that can be improved.

You can become more resilient to life's stressors, more adaptable to change, and, by taking the right approach, you will also get in the shape of your life and increase your energy levels and productivity. The key is to gradually integrate new wellness habits into your routine. By doing so, your ability to tolerate stress will increase, both in daily life and your workouts. We will discuss these wellness habits and how to integrate them into your life in upcoming chapters.

Your stress levels in daily life and your ability to recover will have a direct impact on your capacity to tolerate exercise stress. As we discussed in the previous chapter, it is common to take part in frequent high-intensity workouts in the hope of getting in shape faster. If you are just beginning to exercise, returning after a hiatus or experiencing a lot of stress, this approach may simply add to the load.

EXERCISE

Do you often spend much of the day feeling stressed?

Are you always rushing from one situation to another?

Think about what which parts of your day cause you the most stress and consider your strategies for dealing with them.

High intensity

As my friend and I sat in a busy bar in London watching the Merseyside derby between Liverpool and Everton, we talked about one of Liverpool's young stars, Trent Alexander-Arnold.

An avid Liverpool fan, my friend was worried that the manager was playing Alexander-Arnold too often and was going to burn him out.

It's not unusual to hear people talk about the importance of not overworking a young, talented footballer. Pundits and fans alike will discuss how practice, game time and recovery can be balanced so that the club can get the best out of the player.

When a young player gets overplayed, and their performance begins to decline, or worse, they become injured, conversations about the manager overusing the starlet and risking their long-term career will rage.

But this talk of the young footballer's chances of burning out didn't seem to ring any bells with my friend when it came to how he approached his career and exercise routine.

My friend, who's nearly forty years old and works in a stressful job, regularly takes part in high-intensity workouts without considering burning himself out. He has two young children, so his home life is arguably as busy and stressful as his work life, and his recovery capacity is low. He's under a high amount of stress, his sleep is often disrupted, he drinks a fair amount of alcohol and he works long hours.

No matter how often we speak about the importance of balance in his exercise, he can't seem to pull away from pushing himself to his limits in his workouts. This is common with many high performers I've coached.

I understand the draw – go to the gym, work out intensely and leave. If you're used to being stressed out and working in an intense environment, this type of exercise fits well with the lifestyle.

The release of endorphins and dopamine during high-intensity workouts can become addictive, resulting in people taking part in too many high-intensity workouts without adequate recovery periods.

An endorphin high initially reduces stress and the ability to feel pain. Endorphins are a naturally occurring opiate that act like morphine when released into your brain, and they are addictive.[14] A chemical called endocannabinoids, a natural version of the THC found in marijuana, is also released, and a feel-good buzz follows – but what goes up must come down.[15]

Although most people feel fantastic initially, it often doesn't take long for them to become lethargic; this is the start of the recovery phase. The body adapts to the workout stress and returns to homeostasis.

Unfortunately, instead of relaxing and recovering, many high-performing individuals dive straight into another busy meeting – replacing one stressful environment for another. There's only so much stress one can tolerate.

Just as a footballer will increase the chances of burnout and injury from too many intense matches, you'll suffer the same fate after too many intense workouts. The definition of *intense* is relative to your lifestyle, training experience and ability to recover.

When a footballer enters the twilight of their career – generally by their mid-thirties – they adapt their approach to prolong their career. They understand that they need more rest to stay at their best. They may take more recovery days between matches, and the coach will make sure they rest more regularly.

You're no different from an elite athlete. You need to find the right exercise balance to fit within your routine, lifestyle and training experience. This isn't to say that age should slow down the results you see; you just need to find the right intensity for your needs. This is where balancing your training load is important.

Training load

Think of your training load as the total stress your fitness activities place on your body, generally measured over a week. This includes the frequency, volume (number of repetitions, sets, etc) and intensity of your sessions. The number and intensity of workouts that works for someone else might not work for you. For example, someone who works in a busy, high-stress job and averages 6 hours of sleep won't tolerate the same training load as someone who works fewer hours in a low-stress job and sleeps 8 hours each night. Other factors that impact your recoverability include your age, the quality of your nutrition, how long you've been working out for and your fitness level.

If you consistently push your sessions harder than your capacity to recover, you can end up overreaching.

Overreaching happens as the result of too many intense workouts and not enough recovery. This type of stress can result in a short-term reduction in performance (several days to several weeks).

It may happen after you take part in an excessively intense resistance workout or a long high-intensity interval training (HIIT) session – you'll leave the session feeling wiped out. In the following days, your body will attempt to adapt to the exercise stress. If you train again too soon before fully recovering, and do this consistently over an extended period, you'll be overreaching.

One study showed that more than 30–40 minutes per week of HIIT overloads the nervous system and results in a negative form of stress (distress).[16] Overreaching can be reversed by scheduling adequate rest. However, if you ignore the signs of overreaching, which may include feeling unusually tired or run down, and continue to work out intensely without taking the required recovery periods, it can eventually lead to overtraining syndrome.[17]

Overtraining syndrome is a more severe version of overreaching. It can take several weeks to several months for performance to be restored.

Overtraining can show itself in many ways, including a loss of motivation to work out, excessive tiredness, loss of appetite, and less energy and declined performance when working out. There are also psychological signs, including high emotion, insomnia, and commitment and confidence.

Neither overreaching nor overtraining are beneficial. Although advanced strength trainees can use over-reaching to improve performance, if they follow it with an extended recovery period, it can be detrimental for beginners and intermediate trainees.

Striking the right balance when it comes to your work-out sessions is so important. To achieve this, you need to find the right mix of high-intensity, medium- to high-intensity and lower-intensity sessions for your lifestyle.

Think of high-intensity sessions as pushing yourself to your limit. They require a longer recovery period and should be done only once a week for advanced trainees, unless you're training for an event and are scheduling adequate recovery periods.

A medium- to high-intensity session, such as a typical weight-training session, should make up most of your training load. These sessions will generally require one or two days of recovery. You should leave these sessions feeling like you have worked hard but not wiped out. You should feel buzzed and be looking forward to the next session.

A recovery workout is a lower-intensity session. It will allow you to unwind and switch off. Activities might include doing yoga, walking, cycling and low- to medium-intensity aerobic exercise.

The key is to save your harder workouts for the sessions that are aligned with your fitness goals. For most people who simply want to look and feel better, this would mean saving them for resistance workouts.

As fitness improves and you become more adapted to exercise stressors, you will be able to tolerate a greater training load. Getting in shape takes time and consistent effort. Training intensely in the hope of getting in shape faster can be counterproductive. The focus should be on building good exercise, eating and recovery habits. These will enable you to train harder, recover faster and perform better.

EXERCISE

The next time you work out, consider if you are getting the training load right.

Things to bear in mind:

- Do you feel energised or exhausted after the session?
- Are you excessively tired the following day?

Make a note of how you feel after you train over the next few weeks. If you find yourself excessively tired after or the following day, you may need to adjust the intensity of your workouts.

Balance

We have spoken about how frequent high-intensity workouts can lead to overreaching. It is also important to consider that the definition of 'high intensity' is relative. What is an intense workout to a beginner, may be an easy session for an experienced trainee. Nevertheless, the impact of high-intensity exercise is the same: too many intense workouts without adequate recovery will lead to overreaching, increasing the chance of injury and/or reducing motivation to train. Conversely, not working hard enough will lead to poor results. Finding the right balance is key.

For someone who is just starting out in their fitness journey, the focus should be on building an exercise habit. I have seen countless people try to take part in sessions that are far too intense for their needs. They finish the workout completely wiped out and the thought of returning to the gym is far from appealing.

A 20-minute low-intensity resistance workout is adequate for a beginner. If you want to improve your fitness and you haven't taken part in any cardiovascular training for a while, start by walking. Build up your tolerance to exercise stress, create the right foundations and form an exercise habit. These are the key ingredients for sustainable progress.

If you are currently working out and have plateaued, then it is time to reassess your approach and begin taking a new direction.

Staying in great shape in the twenty-first century is challenging. With improving technology, we have more media fighting for our attention than ever before. At the same time, we have fewer reasons to move and more opportunities to consume high-calorie meals. There is a tendency to focus on quick fixes to counter common problems, but as we have seen, this isn't the right approach for most people.

To look, feel and perform at your best, you need to take a holistic approach. In Part Two, we will look at the nine key areas that will counter the 5Ss and enable you to achieve peak condition.

Key points

- Many people live with high levels of stress for much of the day. There is only so much stress we can tolerate. Adding intense workouts into your day may push you further into a 'recovery debt'.

- Training load is the total stress caused by exercise over a week. The amount of training load you can tolerate is governed by your age, fitness, training experience, diet, stress from other areas of life and sleep.

- It is essential to find the right balance between high-intensity, medium-to-high intensity and recovery sessions to achieve optimal results. The more you train, the better quality of nutrition you consume and the more rest you get, the harder you will be able to push in your sessions. First, build your base and, from there, you'll continue to make progress.

PART TWO
THE PEAK CONDITION METHOD

4

What Is The Peak Condition Method?

The 5Ss are common problems caused by twenty-first-century living. Weight gain, lack of fitness, stiff joints, uncontrolled stress and sleep issues have become more prevalent in modern society.

The nine habits we'll explore in the following chapters are designed to counter the 5Ss. By progressively implementing each habit in your routine, over time, they will help transform how you look, feel and perform.

The nine habits of the Peak Condition Method are split into three core areas: exercise, nutrition and recovery. The principles in this method will help you to adapt to any of life's challenges and maintain a high level of performance.

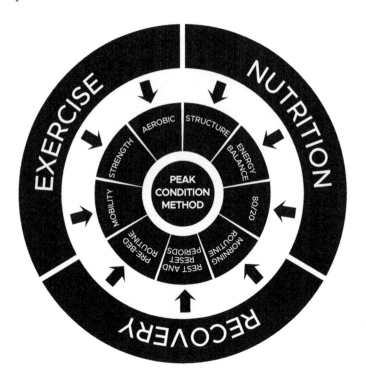

Here's a brief rundown of each of the nine key habits.

Exercise

Mobility base: Improving the strength and control of your joints will enhance your quality of life, exercise performance and longevity.

Strength base: Resistance training will increase lean muscle, bone density and physical strength.

Aerobic base: Low- to medium-intensity cardiovascular training will improve recovery and endurance and will leave you feeling calmer – all crucial in a busy lifestyle.

Nutrition

Structure: A routine that enables you to make healthy food choices consistently will save you time and energy and reduce your chances of making poor choices.

Energy balance: Getting the right balance between the calories you consume and expend will be key to achieving your ideal weight.

80/20: Trying to avoid all treats will be counterproductive and unsustainable. It's important to add treats into your diet, on your terms.

Recovery

Morning routine: The way you start the day has a massive impact on how you perform in it. The better your routine, the more success you'll achieve.

Reset periods: Finding pockets of time during your day to let your brain unwind and recover can be the difference between burning out and thriving in a busy life.

Pre-bed routine: The hours running up to bedtime are crucial when it comes to sleep quality. Following a set routine will significantly increase your likelihood of enjoying a restful night.

This method isn't a radically new concept; it simply focuses on the areas that most busy people over thirty-five who spend most of the day sedentary and who live with a high amount of stress should target.

You have everything you need to reach peak condition

As you introduce the nine habits into your routine, you'll be amazed at the changes you'll experience. Every week will get better. You'll reach a new level of mental and physical performance. The best part is that, before long, it will become your new normal. Having more energy won't be a surprise. You'll get used to looking leaner. Your improved strength and fitness levels will be expected.

You'll raise the bar in terms of what's achievable and expected. You'll soon identify with your new normal.

To get to this point, though, you need to follow a system. You need a strategy.

Getting through the initial phase of building new habits isn't easy. It takes effort, perseverance and an acceptance that it won't all be smooth sailing. Nothing that's worthwhile comes without an element of sacrifice and pushing yourself outside of your comfort zone.

If you're willing to do this, then the process awaits you.

Peak condition scorecard

Before you read on, complete the peak condition scorecard, so you know which areas to focus your attention on first. You can find the scorecard at https://reachyourpeakquiz.com. It takes only 3 minutes to fill out. After you've done so, you'll be sent a customised report indicating where you're already strong and which areas you need to work on the most.

5
Introduction To Exercise

In our daily life, we have fewer reasons to move than ever before. Lifts and escalators have replaced the need to climb stairs. Streaming sites allow us to watch TV for hours on end, and remote controls take away any need to stand up, other than to use the bathroom or make a drink. Doors open automatically, so no need to push. Shopping is done with a click of a button, and many people hire others to do the more physically active domestic jobs, such as gardening and cleaning.

Then there's our work. Research on office-based workers in the UK showed that 71% of the working day was spent doing sedentary activities.[18]

It's common to suffer from stiff, achy joints at a relatively young age, to become out of breath running for a bus and to struggle to hang on to a pull-up bar for more than a few seconds. The sedentary nature of modern society has meant that physical attributes once taken for granted – such as being flexible, strong and aerobically fit – now require work to maintain and improve.

This is why it's so important to build a base of aerobic fitness, mobility and strength. I call this your athletic base. Think of a strong athletic base as the foundation of your physical performance – the platform on which more challenging workouts and physical activity can be performed.

Once you've created a solid base in terms of aerobic exercise, mobility and strength training, every physical activity becomes easier, from playing with young family members to running a marathon. Anything is possible when you create the right foundations.

The three areas that we focus on in exercise are:

- **Mobility base:** A good mobility base involves increasing the strength and control of your joints in multiple planes of motion. Mobility training is an essential ingredient of any workout plan; it will improve your range of motion, relieve achy joints and increase longevity.

- **Strength base:** Building a strength base involves resistance training, such as squats and push-ups.

It will help increase lean muscle, improve bone density and strengthen your range of motion.

- **Aerobic base:** An aerobic base involves training at low to moderate intensities. Fast walking, slow jogging and cycling are examples of this form of exercise, which will improve your recoverability and endurance. It's also less demanding on the nervous system.

We will start by looking at the mobility base.

6
Mobility Base

I've worked out since I was sixteen years old, and I would have started earlier if it hadn't been for my stepdad, who, being a sensible adult, warned me that lifting heavy weights at thirteen wasn't a wise idea. He was a big, well-muscled man, and I was a skinny child with about as much muscle on me as a Twiglet. I had big feet and gangly limbs, which only added insult to injury. I was keen to get into the gym and pump up my puny muscles. In fact, I became obsessed with the idea.

By the time I finally turned sixteen, I was like a raging bull with the red flag of the gym being dangled in front of me. Before long, I became strong for a boy of my age. I loved everything about the gym: the camaraderie, the feeling I got from working out and the results I achieved from the effort I put in. It was a great lesson at a young age: do the hard work and you'll reap the rewards.

I soon went from being a skinny kid to a relatively well-muscled young man. I continued trying to lift as much weight as I could, with all the enthusiasm of youth, utterly unaware of the impact it would have on me in later life.

It wasn't until I was in my late twenties that the effects of my heavy lifting started to show on my body. Looking back, I realise that I skipped the vital foundation stage of working out. This was nobody's fault – it was just how people trained in bodybuilding gyms. You walked in, did a few light warm-up sets and off you went into near-maximal lifts.

Fast-forward twelve years: my back was in pain, as was my left shoulder, my knees throbbed and I often woke up with pain in my neck too. I felt more like a pensioner than a man in my prime.

I was essentially loading my body with weight and trying to perform movements that I couldn't even do without weight. My body compensated by recruiting other muscles, and this led to pain and injury. I'm not alone in this. I know many physical therapists who have practices full of patients with injuries that are the result of poor training techniques and joints unable to handle the load.

Knowing that I had to change my approach to working out, I began to study the fundamentals of human movement and never looked back. I'm now pain free, able to move with more freedom and control at thirty-nine than I could at eighteen and in better shape than ever. This is all down to practising movement daily and finding balance in my training.

We'll look at two strategies to maintain joint health and improve range of motion. First, though, let's explore one of the main causes of stiff joints and the importance of making exercise choices which match your movement capacity.

Stiff joints

The body needs movement. For much of human evolution we climbed, crawled and spent long periods walking. We also spent long periods being sedentary, but the balance between the two was right. Fast-forward to the twenty-first century, and that balance has disappeared, with negative consequences for our joint health.

Studies have shown that living a sedentary lifestyle can increase the chances of suffering from orthopaedic problems such as lower back and knee pain.[19] It may manifest initially as a feeling of stiffness or tightness, but over time, this turns into pain.

The prevalence of lower back and neck pain is rising in the UK, according to research from the British

Chiropractic Association. Some 65% of people surveyed reported experiencing back or neck ache once a month, while 49% of people surveyed said they suffered from back or neck ache weekly. Nearly half (45%) reported sitting still for long periods of time as a trigger for their pain.[20]

When we spend long periods in the same position, such as sitting down, our central nervous system (CNS), which controls movement, learns that this is how the body is primarily used. The CNS then essentially adjusts movement capacity to match what it perceives we need. The result is dysfunctional joints that feel stiff and restricted when we move them in certain positions.

Your joints are continuously communicating with your CNS in a process called afferent feedback. For a joint to function optimally, it must have good motion. This allows for efficient communication with the nervous system. A restricted joint communicates poorly with the nervous system.[21]

Imagine being upstairs in your house with the doors closed and your partner shouting from downstairs. You'd likely struggle to hear what they were saying. The closer you are, the clearer the words become. In the communication between the CNS and a joint, the words become muffled when a joint is dysfunctional, resulting in inefficient movement.

It is common for someone to begin exercising in the hope that it will reduce stiff and achy joints, but it can make the problem worse if not approached in the right way. The primary way to counter a sedentary life is by integrating a mobility practice into your routine and choosing exercises that suit your movement capacity. Avoid taking part in workouts that are ill-suited to your needs, as this can result in pain and ultimately injury.

Dynamic workouts

There are many workouts that involve a combination of dynamic body-weight exercises, such as burpees and squat jumps, and resistance exercises, performed with high repetitions and little rest between sets. Dynamic exercises generally involve explosive movements and are designed to generate power.

The dynamic nature of the exercises can be ill-suited to much of the general public, with many people not having the prerequisite strength or mobility to perform the activities prescribed. When technical exercises are performed with high repetitions and minimal recovery, technique is inevitably impacted.

It's unwise for anyone who suffers from stiff joints and sits for much of the day to do these types of workouts.

High repetitions + dynamic exercise + poor technique = increased chance of injury

It isn't only dynamic exercises that can cause injury, but heavy resistance training performed with poor technique. It is important to choose exercises that you can do with good form and pain free. Then focus on improving your joint mobility and, with it, the number of exercises you can perform.

The aim when doing mobility training is to prepare your joints to withstand stress in multiple planes of motion, improve the body's performance, reduce the chance of injury and increase longevity.

Mobility is perhaps the most fundamental quality in fitness. When movement is restricted, your ability to take part in certain activities will be limited.

You'll also be restricted in the number of exercises you can perform. Although you can always find alternative exercises, fundamentally, we're training to improve the quality of our lives and the performance of our bodies. Issues such as lower back pain may stop you from taking part in activities such as playing with a young family member or being able to pick something up off the floor.

The long-term health of your joints is dependent on their being taken through a full range of motion, regularly. For example, in parts of Southeast Asia, such as Thailand, it's common to see senior citizens waiting for buses in a deep squat position – they don't think anything of it; it's just something they've always been able to do. Every time they wait for a bus, they sit in that position, so they maintain that range of motion. If they didn't do this regularly, they'd lose it.

If you don't use it, you'll lose it.

The good news is you can regain lost range of motion. The secret is to add dedicated mobility training into your training programme and invest time into moving your joints regularly.

Flexibility and mobility

Think of mobility training as strength training for your joints. Just as you need to add stress into your muscles to allow them to adapt and become stronger, you need to do the same with your joints. When it comes to your joints, there are two main areas of focus – flexibility and mobility.

Flexibility is about lengthening your muscles passively. Imagine bending over to touch your toes – this is a passive stretch.

Mobility is about the control and strength of your joints through the full range of motion – imagine touching your toes and picking up an object from the floor. Your mobility is your active range of motion.

If your joints have become 'tight', you'll need to increase both flexibility and mobility.

The aim is to add controlled resistance into your joints in different positions, so they know how to act in each one. Controlled resistance will strengthen your joints in a wider range of motion, improving how they function and making them more durable. You'll also be stronger when working out. If you have a limited range of motion, you are essentially tighter and weaker in certain ranges.

The difference between someone who rolls their ankle and gets ligament damage and someone who walks away without any injury is often down to the strength and control in that range of motion. The better your mobility, the better you function as a human.

If you want to improve your physical performance, focusing on improving joint mobility is an absolute must. One of the most effective ways to improve the control of your movement is by performing joint rotations.

Joint rotations

You may have seen older people rotate their joints as a type of stretch. Well, they're on the right track.

Joint rotations are simple but highly effective in terms of improving joint health.

I learned about joint rotations, or controlled articular rotations (CARS), in a seminar by world-renowned chiropractor Dr Andreo Spina.[22] I have included them in my own routine and programmed them into clients' plans ever since.

The rotations involve taking each of your major joints through a full range of circular motion. This increases blood flow, sending nutrients and lubrication to the joint and improving the communication with your CNS, so it understands where your joint is in space (this is called proprioception).

It's important to move the joint independently of other areas of your body. Often, when we move one limb, the body compensates by recruiting other limbs to aid the movement and, over time, the brain will automatically make everything move as one. This can lead to unhealthy joints due to a lack of blood flow to that joint and a reduced ability to clear metabolic waste. Aim to take each joint through its greatest range of motion without compensating by moving any other part of your body.

It's a good practice to add rotations to your morning routine so you essentially warm up and prepare your joints for the demands of the upcoming day. It's also important to stand up, move around and rotate your joints whenever possible. Even moving just one joint will be beneficial. This will reduce the impact of a sedentary lifestyle and keep your joints healthy. I call this process 'exercise snacking'.

When the day is in full flow, it's easy to forget to stand up and move around, so I set myself an alarm to remind me to get up and move. Over time, exercise snacking will become a habit.

Joint rotations fundamentally focus on improving joint control; if you're stiff and feel as if your joints are restricted, more prolonged passive stretching will be required.

EXERCISE

Think about how you could find five minutes to practise joint rotations each day.

Passive stretching

Holding a passive stretch can be relaxing – and relaxation is precisely what you're trying to achieve. When you are stretching, you are not lengthening muscle fibres; you are essentially trying to convince your nervous system to allow you to access more range of motion.

Think of it in this context: if your nervous system doesn't feel confident that you'll be able to move into a position without becoming injured or being able to move out of it, something called your stretch reflex will kick in and stop you from performing that movement. An example of this is bending down to grab an object off the floor but not being able to reach it. Your stretch reflex is activated to protect you from hurting your back or getting stuck in the position.

The aim is to delay that stretch reflex, so it kicks in later than it currently does. Physiologically, when you're holding a stretch, you're trying to alter your stretch tolerance so that you gain greater range of motion in your joints. You can do this by holding a passive stretch for more than 2 minutes. While performing the stretch, take deep, diaphragmatic breaths to relax your nervous system and, in turn, allow you to move deeper into the stretch. Don't hold your breath or take shallow breaths.

It's important to keep in mind that flexibility without control over that range is just as dangerous as poor flexibility in itself. Imagine being about to move your arm into the air without any resistance, but then someone threw a ball quickly at you and you had to catch the ball dynamically with your arms outstretched overhead; if you didn't have strength in that position, you might get injured.

This is why doing resisted mobility training and flexibility training is essential. The idea is to stretch the joint so that you gain more movement and then strengthen it so that you can consolidate that newly acquired range of motion. You can achieve this by putting controlled resistance into the joint through the full range, such as when doing resistance training. This will build resilient and healthy joints.

For best results, repeat this process multiple times each week, and over time you'll notice your range of motion increasing. The benefits will be worth it. Your body will become more robust and functional.

Key points

- Long periods spent in the same position signal to the nervous system that this is the primary use of the body and it will reduce range of motion, leaving you feeling stiff and tight.

- To counter this problem, we need to move our joints through a full range of motion. Aim to stand up regularly and rotate each major joint, as well as start the day with joint rotations.

- To increase flexibility, aim to hold a stretch for 2 minutes or more. This will increase the joint's pliability. Consolidate it by doing controlled strength training through a full range of motion.

FREE GIFT

Download your free joint rotation plan and a demonstration of how to passively stretch and strengthen the range at www.pathtopeakcondition .com/freegift

7
Strength Base

Being strong is important: we need strong muscles, strong joints, strong bones and strong immune systems, among others. Strength training will help with each of these and much more. It is fundamental to our performance, overall health and quality of life. It can give us confidence in our ability to perform everyday tasks and take on physical challenges. It can also counter some of the physical decline that we experience as we age.

As we age, muscle mass begins to decline, in a process called sarcopenia. A young male's body weight, for example, will generally be made up of 50% muscle mass, but this will steadily decline after the age of thirty, and by the time he's in his mid-seventies, he will have lost 25% of his lean muscle. The rate is shown to accelerate between the ages of forty and sixty.[23]

We can consolidate and even increase muscle mass by performing resistance training throughout life. According to data published in *Medicine and Science in Sports and Exercise*, men between the ages of fifty and eighty-three who performed progressive resistance training increased their lean body mass by about 1 kg.[24]

A decline in muscle mass is just one impact on the musculoskeletal system caused by aging. Bone is a living tissue and is continuously broken down and rebuilt. Up to the age of around twenty-five, the rebuild is quicker than the breakdown, so bone density increases. The rates of breakdown and repair stay relatively stable until the age of about fifty, when bone breakdown begins to outpace bone formation and bones begins to weaken. In the UK, 3 million people suffer from osteoporosis (a weakening of bones).[25] Weakened bones break more easily. Estimates suggest that 50% of women over the age of fifty and 20% of men will suffer a fracture related to osteoporosis.[26]

You can reduce this decline by taking part in progressive resistance training. By adding stress to the bones, you will increase bone density, and this can reduce the risk of osteoporosis.[27] The need to take part in resistance training is more important than ever before due to the sedentary nature of modern living. It is essential to maintain a healthy and robust body.

Creating solid foundations and progressing at the right pace will ensure you get the most from your resistance workouts. We will look at this in more detail in this chapter.

DOMS

At about the midpoint of my travels in my twenties, I treated myself to a nice hotel (there had been some bad ones along the way!). The hotel had a plush fitness centre, and as soon as I entered the gym, all my old excitement flooded back.

I hadn't worked out with resistance for nearly a year, but I ignored that fact and set about trying to replicate the sort of workout that I would have done before starting my travels. I was still able to lift a decent amount of weight, and I pushed myself while enjoying the buzz of endorphins that I'd missed so much. I was happy with my efforts and walked away from my workout feeling tired but good about myself – until I woke up the next day.

As soon as I opened my eyes, I knew I was in trouble. My body felt heavy; standing up and shuffling to the shower required a substantial effort. As the day progressed, I began feeling a lot like the Tin Man from the *Wizard of Oz*. My arms were bent at a 90-degree angle, and simple tasks such as lowering myself to the toilet seat felt like torture. Pain was just one of the side effects.

I was also extremely tired and groggy. I had no energy. Mentally and physically, I felt worn out.

I'd ignored the advice that I'd offered to others countless times before and completely overdone it. I'd worked out much harder than I needed to.

The pain I was feeling is called delayed onset muscle soreness (DOMS). It's the ache that you feel when your muscles work harder than they're used to or in a different way. DOMS is believed to be caused by microscopic damage to the muscle. As your body repairs itself, it increases in strength and lean muscle to better tolerate the stressor the next time around.

Although uncomfortable, DOMS is an expected by-product of a hard workout, and a positive training effect, but not in this severity. My uncomfortable experience lasted for about seven days. If I'd wanted to work out again that week, I would have struggled to. I was in far too much pain and lacked motivation to do anything.

If I hadn't known that the aching and tiredness was my fault for working out too intensely, I might have been put off training. I've spoken to people who genuinely believed they'd injured themselves because their DOMS was so bad.

Pain is often seen as the marker of a good workout, but it shouldn't be. Pushing yourself so hard that you struggle to move for a week, let alone exercise, is counterproductive. All the good work done in the session will be undone because the recovery period will be too long. Working out effectively is about improving performance and progress week on week. If you go too hard in each session, this will be difficult to achieve.

Technique

Go into most gyms and you'll see people lifting weights with poor technique. Generally, this means they're using more weight than they can control and because of this, they need to create momentum to move the weight around.

There's a common misconception that more resistance is best to see progress, but more weight is often about boosting the ego rather than improving performance.

When I began resistance training, I wanted to lift as much weight as possible. I wore straps around my knees and a weight belt around my waist when squatting in the hope that I could handle more weight. In truth, I was more concerned about looking strong than I was about my technique.

If your goal is to become a powerlifter, it's obviously important to lift as much weight as possible, but if you simply want to progress your training and increase lean muscle, it's much wiser to reduce the weight slightly and focus on executing the exercise with correct form.

This is where many people go wrong. They lift much heavier weight than they need to, putting unnecessary pressure on their joints, causing excessive DOMS following the workout and reducing their capacity to recover from the session.

Mastering technique is essential when new to resistance training. Sacrificing form to lift more weight will impact your progress in the longer term.

Think of elite tennis players. They will continuously practise their serve, forehand and backhand, so they can improve how they strike a ball. In doing so, they will be able to generate more power, hit the ball with more accuracy and enhance their performance.

Whichever stage of your resistance training journey you are on, it is essential to continue to focus on exercise execution. You will improve neuromuscular coordination and become faster, stronger and more efficient at performing the movement. Your technique is also a key driver to build lean muscle. Manipulating the speed of your repetitions and focusing on creating tension during a working set are essential to stimulate growth of lean muscle mass, which is fundamental to weight management and our immune system.

There are three mechanisms to induce lean muscle growth.[28] The first is mechanical tension.

Mechanical tension

Mechanical tension essentially means lifting weight through a full range of motion. That can be your body weight or an external load. The aim is to execute each repetition with good form and to focus on creating tension in the muscle or region of muscles you're targeting. It's often called the 'mind–muscle connection'.

Let's use the example of doing a push-up. Imagine as you're lowering yourself to the floor that you're resisting and therefore creating tension. As you push away, you're slowly contracting the muscle, adding force towards and away from the floor.

The more time spent under load, the more mechanical tension you'll experience. It's a fundamental training mechanism to improve strength and lean muscle. However, it's only one of a number of ways to manipulate technique. Metabolic stress is another.

Metabolic stress

Metabolic stress is a form of training where you perform more repetitions with a shorter recovery to generate a burning sensation, also known as a pump.

Using moderate to light weight will allow you to achieve more repetitions, and this will cause an anabolic effect, increasing the hormonal response and resulting in muscle growth.[29] Just because you're doing more repetitions, though, it doesn't mean you need more momentum. While the speed of the movement can increase, tension is still essential during this form of training.

One of the benefits of doing more repetitions is that your muscle is under load for longer; this increases the volume your muscle has to tolerate – one of the primary ways to stimulate muscle growth. Another way to achieve this is by using a technique called muscle damage.

Muscle damage

Muscle damage has been caused by the time a muscle is under tension. The most muscle damage occurs when performing the eccentric (downward) phase of the movement slowly.

Muscle damage is a highly effective way to increase lean muscle,[30] but be warned: it can cause severe DOMS. I wouldn't advise a beginner to try this form of training.

Technique is an important aspect of resistance training. Well-executed repetitions can be the difference between progressing at a fast rate or plateauing and increasing the chance of injury.

Progressive overload

To improve performance and increase lean muscle, you need to overload your body's ability to tolerate stress. During the recovery period, your body will adapt by increasing its capacity to handle the stressor the next time around. In each workout that follows, you repeat this process – train to a level where you force your body into an adaptive response.

Think of a martial artist who often gets kicked in their shins. They need to strengthen their shins so they can withstand a hard leg kick the next time they fight, and they do this by hitting their shins with a plank of wood time and again, causing microscopic damage. They understand that unless they build up tolerance to that stressor and make their shins stronger, they risk injury.

In fitness, this theory is called progressive overload, and it's pivotal to improving your body's performance.

The aim when working out is to administer just the right amount of stress into your body in the form of resistance training, followed by adequate recovery. No more, no less. In doing so, you force your muscle to become bigger and stronger. Every time you work out, you'll need to challenge your body slightly more than you did in your previous workout to force an adaptative response.

If you're new to resistance training or have taken a sustained hiatus, your tolerance to exercise stress will be lower than that of someone who has worked out consistently for a long time.

Just as your chronological age is how long you've been alive, your training age is the amount of time you've spent doing a particular activity or type of training. If you've been doing resistance training regularly for fifteen years, you'll have a training age of fifteen; if you're new to resistance training, your training age will be close to zero.

Your training age will have a significant impact on how much stress you can tolerate from a workout. Many trainees develop well as beginners. Since the body hasn't been subjected to resistance training before, muscle growth and strength increase rapidly. This is one of the main reasons that resistance training should be started slowly – it takes less stress for the body to become overwhelmed, and the chances of overreaching increase.

You can overload your body in several ways:

- Increase the load – progressively add weight

- Increase the volume – add reps or sets to your workouts

- Decrease the rest period – reduce the amount of rest between sets

- Increase the number of workouts in a week

- Increase the complexity of the workout – supersets (two exercises for different muscle groups, performed back-to-back) compound sets (two exercises from the same muscle group performed back-to-back), etc

- Increase the duration of the workout – time spent training

The progressive overload principle can also be applied to your cardiovascular and mobility workouts to create stronger and more resilient joints, and improve your aerobic metabolism and the cardiorespiratory system. In fact, progressive overload can be used to improve each of the nine habits in this book to ensure you are continuously improving your health and well-being.

The most effective way to implement progressive overload into your workouts is by following a training cycle.

Training cycle

A training cycle is a structured plan for your upcoming workouts and can be split into macro-, meso- and micro-cycles. A macro-cycle is generally based over a year and takes into account competitions and events. A meso-cycle typically lasts one month. A micro-cycle usually lasts seven days. For most people, focusing on the upcoming month will be enough.

The plan doesn't have to be complicated or in-depth but should include what you'll do in each session for the upcoming week. It's best to use the same training programme for three to six weeks, so you can make steady improvements each week.

I prefer changing my training plan every calendar month. This duration is long enough to stay focused but not so long that the workouts become boring.

For the first few weeks of a training phase, you'll notice muscle and strength gains, but the increased muscle will mainly come from muscle damage-induced swelling and the increased strength will mostly be from neural adaptation (essentially, your brain and body learning the exercises).[31] After this point, you'll see true strength and muscle gains, which are two of the primary goals of resistance training.[32]

Stopping the training phase early and changing exercises will simply mean you'll need to go through the learning phase again, and much of the soreness that comes with beginning a new training plan.

By following a structured plan over several weeks, you'll also be able to progress the workout week on week and force an adaptive response; this is progressive overload in action. If you continue using the same plan for too long, however, your body will adapt to the stressor and the workout will become less effective. In turn, your progress will begin to slow.

At this stage, it's important to remember that the definition of intensity is relative. If you're just beginning to work out, you'll need to do much less than a seasoned trainee.

The best way to assess if you're getting the intensity right to force an adaptation is to measure the rate of perceived exertion (RPE).

RPE

RPE means how hard you are working. It was first conceived by Gunnar Borg in 1970 to assess the intensity of endurance training using a scale of 6–20.[33] Although effective for aerobic exercise, this scale didn't transfer as well to resistance training due to the definition of 'max effort'.

Since then, it has been modified for resistance training by Mike Tuchscherer, using reps in reserve at the end of a working set.[34] The effectiveness of this approach has been validated in various studies.[35]

I use the below scale to assess how many reps in reserve I have during a working set:

10 – no more reps left in the tank

9 – 1 rep left

8 – 2 reps left

7 – 3 reps left

6 – 4 reps left

5 – 5 reps left

4 or below – recovery session

For most training sessions, I recommend staying between 7 and 8 on the scale. This is the optimal level of stress, where your body is forced into an adaptive response but your ability to recover from the session isn't affected.[36]

If your RPE is often at 6 or below, you may not be working out hard enough to progress. At this point, you should increase the effort level – that is, unless you're doing a recovery session (4 or below). If you continuously creep up to 9 or 10, you may be training too hard.

It is important to note that people often think they are working harder than they are. It is not uncommon for someone to say that their workout was a 7–8 on the RPE scale when they were really at a 5–6. A 10 out of 10 on the scale means you have pushed yourself to complete failure and are unable to do any more repetitions. Working towards a 7–8 on the scale means that you are two to three reps from complete failure. That is still working incredibly hard, and this level of intensity is required to force the body to adapt and improve.[37]

At the beginning of a new resistance training phase, reduce the RPE slightly and stop three or four reps below complete failure on the first session. If you push too hard at the beginning of a training phase, it will be harder to progress the workout, and you may even go back over the period. Remember, the aim is to work slightly harder each workout to force an adaptive response.

It's important to listen to your body and look out for signs that you need to reduce the intensity of your workouts. This is called autoregulation.

Autoregulation

It can be difficult to differentiate between feeling tired and being lazy. Working out intensely when exhausted can leave you feeling worse than when you began, which is unproductive.

You may feel lazy if you reduce the effort level of your training, but really, you're simply adapting your workout to match your energy level so that you get the most from it without burning yourself out. This is where autoregulation comes in.

Autoregulation enables you to adjust your training workload before the session if you feel extremely tired or during it if you are struggling to hit the normal levels you have come to expect.

At the beginning of each workout, rate how you feel on a scale of 1 to 10.

A rating below 5 will mean that you had to drag yourself out of bed that morning and needed coffee to get through the day.

A rating of 5 to 7 will mean you're functioning well but not quite up to your normal standard. You may feel foggy and slightly demotivated.

A rating of 8 to 10 means you feel good and full of energy.

If you're below 5, take a rest day or replace your planned workout with a recovery session. If you're at 5 or above, continue with the session while using RPE to adjust your workload to how you feel.

If you rated yourself between 5 and 7 at the beginning of the session but feel energised during it, then continue as usual. If you're still not functioning at your normal standard, reduce the intensity of your workout by giving yourself more rest between sets or doing fewer total sets.

Autoregulation is a key part of managing and progressing your workouts. Training hard if you haven't had enough recovery will simply push you further into 'recovery debt'. If you're stressed out, struggle to get good-quality sleep and/or eat a highly processed diet, your ability to recover will be impacted. Train to how you feel on a given day – you'll experience better results for it.

It's important to note that autoregulation does come with its problems. It is not always easy to judge how hard you should train based on how you feel. If you're someone who enjoys pushing it to the limit, you may ignore the signs of fatigue and could end up with injuries and/or overtraining. If you're prone to taking it easy, you may not work hard enough to cause an adaptive response and progress may stall.

It may help to consider how your performance in the workout stands up to your previous workouts in the programme. If you're struggling to lift the same weight or achieve the same numbers of sets, you may need to drop the effort level by taking more rest or making the session slightly shorter. Alternatively, it may be time to step up the effort level if you're finding the workout too easy.

Remember, your workout is only as good as your ability to recover from it. Training hard when you're tired, just because you have a session planned, can be detrimental to your progress and well-being.

Focusing on getting the intensity of your training right will enable you to continuously improve your physical capacity.

EXERCISE

Next time you work out, rate your energy level from 1 to 10 and adapt your session to how you feel on that day.

Continue doing this and you'll begin to develop a better understanding of how to adapt your training to match your energy and recoverability.

Key points

- When you begin a resistance programme, the priority is to focus on technique and implement progressive overload. This will give you a good foundation from which to work.

- Follow a structured training plan for a calendar month with the aim of progressing your workouts week on week by increasing the weight or number of repetitions or sets.

- Be aware that you can push too hard and overtrain. Adapt your workouts to how you feel by giving your energy level a rating from 1 to 10 before your workout, and adjust your intensity during the session using RPE. You'll see better results for it.

8
Aerobic Base

There is much debate surrounding which is a more beneficial modality of cardiovascular exercise – HIIT or lower-intensity aerobic training.

The truth is that neither is better or worse; what works best for you simply depends on your goals, fitness level, training experience and recoverability.

HIIT predominantly uses the anaerobic system and lower-intensity cardiovascular exercise uses predominantly the aerobic system. Let's look at the energy systems in more detail.

The human body has three central energy systems which fuel all our activity – phosphocreatine, anaerobic and aerobic. Think of an energy system as your body's primary way of transforming food into energy. Cells can use this energy for activities such as walking, running and weightlifting. Your body breaks down the food source into smaller molecules – protein to amino acids, carbohydrates to glycogen and fat to triglycerides. Amino acids are rarely used as a source of energy for physical activity when sufficient glycogen and triglycerides are available. These molecules need to be converted into adenosine triphosphate (ATP).

The first burst of energy you get when you work out, which lasts for about 10–20 seconds, is created by phosphocreatine, also known as creatine phosphate. It generates ATP for brief, intense bursts of effort. This energy system takes much longer than the others to recharge.

Phosphocreatine will be the main energy system in use during a 100-metre sprint.

Second to kick in is the anaerobic system, which generates ATP without oxygen. Most of this energy comes from the glycogen stored in your muscles and the glucose in your blood. This system is associated with high-intensity, sugar-burning activities that last more than 20 seconds but less than 2 minutes. The anaerobic system will be the main one in use during a 400-metre race.

The aerobic system primarily uses oxygen and is associated with fatigue-free, fat-burning activities. It generates ATP during workouts lasting more than 2 minutes, and it relies mainly on fat as fuel. The aerobic system is primarily used during longer runs, such as 5,000- and 10,000-metre races.[38]

Deciding whether HIIT or lower-intensity aerobic exercise is best suited to your training needs will have a big impact on the results you see. We will look at both in this chapter.

High-intensity anaerobic exercise

HIIT is everywhere. You'll find free classes on social media, and gym timetables are full of variations that will quickly elevate your heart rate.

HIIT involves short bursts of intense activity followed by an active recovery. The main aim of HIIT is to raise the heart rate to an anaerobic state – 85% or more of maximum heart rate (MHR) – followed by active recovery, allowing the heart to return to an aerobic state, which is between 50% and 70% MHR. Heart rate is only one measure. Effort level and power output – the amount of intensity or velocity produced per unit time – are other good markers.

HIIT is best suited to being performed on a stationary apparatus such as a bike, treadmill or versa climber, enabling you to produce high, sustained power output.

If you are unable to maintain the desired intensity or velocity, you are likely not allowing sufficient recovery or your intervals are too long.

This could mean you follow a work-to-rest ratio of one work to four times recovery, but it depends on your fitness level.

Many HIIT classes don't allow for enough recovery to ensure the individual can hit the required power output. I can testify that it's challenging to instruct a class full of different fitness levels where 30 seconds of maximum effort is followed by 2 minutes of active recovery. The participants get bored.

The activity essentially becomes an extended intense cardio session. The heart rate remains elevated in an anaerobic zone. The participants cannot either hit the required power output or allow their heart rate to return to the aerobic zone because they don't have enough recovery time. This makes the session highly demanding on the nervous system, leaving participants feeling burnt out and adding a substantial amount of training load. That is why I now recommend that most people do not take part in this type of HIIT class.

To get the most out of your HIIT session, it is best to keep the workout short and focus on near-maximum effort, followed by a long-enough rest period which enables you to recover sufficiently to achieve the same power output the next time around. Avoid workouts that incorporate body-weight plyometric exercises that require you to jump up and down, such as burpees and squat jumps, with minimal rest periods. These workouts will do little more than increase your chances of injury, and it will be nigh on impossible to hit the desired effort level due to the nature of the exercises.

If incorporated as part of a structured plan with adequate recovery following the session, HIIT can be a great addition to your training schedule when you have a strong aerobic base, but it's not necessary for someone who is just starting an exercise regime. It should be included in your plan only when you're at the intermediate to advanced stage of your exercise journey and you have implemented the other strategies in this book to improve recoverability.

If you're just starting out and building an aerobic base, performing low- to medium-intensity cardiovascular training is essential. Although often seen as the less attractive alternative to anaerobic exercise, aerobic exercise is an excellent training modality for busy people.

Aerobic training

Aerobic exercise is a less demanding alternative to anaerobic training. It's the perfect foil for more intense workouts. Low- to moderate-intensity activities such as brisk walking, light jogging and cycling fall into the bracket of aerobic exercise.

Low-intensity cardio has many benefits, including improved cardiovascular function, deeper, more restful sleep, and less stress and anxiety.[39] A strong aerobic energy system can help you recover more quickly from intense bouts of exercise and between training sessions.[40]

It's common for the heart rate to quickly increase to an anaerobic zone during cardiovascular exercise. By improving the aerobic system, you'll stay in your aerobic zone longer and improve endurance. Not only that, but you'll also return to your aerobic system faster after periods of high-intensity (anaerobic) exercise and increase the flow of oxygen, blood and nutrients to the muscles. That means you'll recover more quickly between resistance exercises and during interval training.[41]

If you have poor aerobic development, you'll have the capacity to perform only a few hard intervals or intense sets before fatigue sets in – the quality of the workout will decline as a result.

Aerobic heart rate zone 2 activities, which will put you between 60% and 70% MHR, will increase your work capacity and recovery speed. You'll burn predominantly fat while in this heart rate zone. There are five zones, and they are based on your heart rate. Zone 1 is 50–60% MHR and Zone 5 is 90–100% MHR.

Aerobic exercise also improves the body's ability to use and mobilise fat. A study at Duke University, which was the largest trial of its kind, measured how different forms of exercise improved body composition. It was found that aerobic exercise was the best for burning fat.[42]

Initially, it may feel as if you're not doing enough when training at this relatively low intensity. You may want to increase the intensity of the workout, but persevere. Before long, your pace will quicken at that same heart rate.

Depending on your starting point, 15–20 minutes of moderate-intensity cardiovascular exercise will improve your fitness. As you progress, aim to increase the frequency and duration until you achieve a minimum of two or three 30-minute sessions of cardiovascular training each week.

Brisk walking will likely be enough for you to enter aerobic zone 2, especially if you're currently inactive. Again, though, don't worry – your aerobic base will improve fast.

Aerobic training isn't just beneficial to your physical health but also to your mental health.

Numerous studies have shown that moderate-intensity aerobic exercise improves the parasympathetic nervous response.[43] This is the calm cousin of fight or flight – rest and digest.

I use aerobic exercise to improve my endurance and recover from an intense workday, allowing my mind to switch gears. No matter what mindset I take into the session, I'll come out of it feeling positive. I choose relaxing music and let my mind wander. Any stress of the day is soon replaced by an upbeat mood. This is quite different from when I do high-intensity cardio sessions, where, due to the intensity, I switch off and concentrate only on the workout itself.

I see intense workouts as a way to switch off, while lower-intensity workouts are a way to sort out my thoughts and problem-solve. They both have benefits, but in a world full of stress, it's important to use low-intensity exercise as a strategy to recover.

One of the best ways to improve your aerobic capacity is to use low-intensity interval training (LIIT).

EXERCISE

Next time you do a cardio session, track your heart rate using a smartwatch or heart rate monitor. Look at how quickly your heart rate increases compared to your exercise intensity. The longer you stay in your aerobic zone, the better your aerobic base.

LIIT

As you begin an aerobic exercise routine, you may notice that your heart rate quickly elevates, or you may struggle to keep going for long periods. This is where LIIT comes in.

LIIT is similar to HIIT in that it involves intervals of increased intensity followed by periods of lower intensity. The main difference is that LIIT is much lower in its overall intensity. For example, HIIT may combine a period of sprinting with a slow jog to recover, whereas LIIT will combine a slow jog with walking.

LIIT is perfect for anyone who has a low aerobic capacity – those just starting cardiovascular training or returning after a long hiatus, for instance. If you struggle to run for an extended period, this modality of aerobic exercise will work well for you.

As discussed, if your aerobic system is underdeveloped, you may quickly enter your anaerobic zone even when going relatively slowly. Using a heart rate monitor or smartwatch, determine when your heart rate enters the anaerobic zone and then reduce your speed. This may involve transitioning between a slow jog and walking. Don't overthink this. If you feel like you are exerting yourself but can still hold a conversation, you are likely in the right heart-rate zone.

Before long, you'll be able to stay in your aerobic zone for longer intervals of cardiovascular exercise. Your speed and endurance will increase, as will your rate of recovery.

Aerobic training can be used as a recovery workout to supplement resistance training and more intense sessions. Not only will you get an abundance of physiological benefits, but you'll also get crucial mental downtime away from the stressors of life – it's an essential element of your exercise schedule.

Key points

- Although popular, most high-intensity classes are too long and don't allow enough recovery time between intervals to work both the anaerobic and aerobic energy systems.

- Aerobic exercise offers a lower-intensity alternative. It will improve your ability to recover, use predominantly fat as energy and leave you feeling calmer.

- To build up your aerobic base, start by doing brisk walks and then transfer into LIIT, moving from slow jogs and walking. Your aerobic capacity will quickly improve.

We've now looked at how to build a strong athletic base. As you build a base of aerobic fitness, mobility and strength, every physical activity will become easier. You'll move with more freedom, recover faster, improve your physical performance and gain more confidence in your body.

It's essential to focus on building the right foundations before moving on to more intense workouts. Treat it as an integral part of your training schedule. The fact is, without a strong base, you'll never become the best athletic version of yourself. Of course, your athletic base is just one element when it comes to achieving peak condition.

Next, we'll look at how to fuel your body.

9
Introduction To Nutrition

We can order fast food straight to our doorstep. High streets are full of takeaways, and food seems to be advertised everywhere. The options available have never been so abundant, and they're harder than ever to ignore.

Fast food is developed to taste good. Manufacturers have tuned in to our innate drive to eat calorie-rich food. The high sodium and sugar content may not be healthy, but it sure is appealing to the taste buds. The combination of fats, gums, starches, emulsifiers and stabilisers in processed food creates the sensation of a meal that melts in your mouth. The perfect balance of crunchiness and chewiness, combined with saltiness, sugariness and fattiness, can be hard to resist. Fast food is designed to be hyperpalatable, and it can be addictive, leaving us wanting more.

Hyperpalatable food overrides the brain's reward neurocircuitry and essentially switches off the 'stop eating' signal. Researchers have found that 'the synergy between key ingredients in a food creates an artificially enhanced palatability experience that is greater than any key ingredient would produce alone'. These foods combined either fat and sodium, such as bacon; fat and simple sugars, such as cookies; or carbohydrates and sodium, such as popcorn.[44]

Food scientists study mouthfeel to perfectly balance the density and dryness, crunchiness and chewiness of food. Once these factors are combined with an appealing taste and smell, the food will be too good to resist.

Not only is fast food hard to resist, but we are being served more of it. A study which looked at portion sizes in the United States, found that 'most marketplace portions exceed standard serving sizes by at least a factor of two and sometimes eight-fold. Portions have increased over time; those offered by fast-food chains, for example, often are two to five times larger than the original size.'[45] Although this obviously doesn't mean we need to eat more food, it is hard not to. Another study showed that when the portion size was larger, participants consumed 16% more food.[46]

With the odds seemingly stacked against us, it's no surprise that obesity numbers are at an all-time high and rising. The diet culture is clearly not working, and there are many reasons why, but a few are glaringly obvious. Many diets focus solely on reductionism instead of behavioural change. They'll typically involve either drastically reducing calorie intake or reducing a macronutrient, such as fat or carbohydrates.

When you consider the facts that processed food is often hyperpalatable, and that food cravings increase when restricting calorie intake, it is no wonder that dieting is hard to sustain.

Diets create a short-term mindset instead of encouraging you to look longer term. The fact is that you're going to be eating for the rest of your life, so your focus should be on adapting your eating habits, to maintain a healthy weight and supply your body with what it needs to perform at its best.

There are, three fundamental principles to follow to achieve this balance:

- **Structure:** This is crucial to ensure you remain consistent with your food choices and are able to plan ahead. The goal is to create healthy eating habits which become second nature. This won't happen without planning and structure.

- **Energy balance:** Finding the right energy balance is fundamental in the journey to achieve your aesthetic goals.

- **80/20:** A sustainable diet needs to have space for treats alongside food that is nutritious and satisfying. Aim for 80% of your calorie intake to be real, whole food and save 20% for treats.

There's no need for guesswork. You simply need to adjust your diet so that it's well rounded and matches your routine and calorie requirements. Dieting doesn't lead to long-term weight loss; changing your eating habits does. This is why creating structure is essential.

10
Structure

In the City of London at lunchtime you will see people rushing around to grab a quick bite to eat. There is an abundance of food options to choose from, but limited time to decide.

Making a quick food decision increases the chances of choosing badly. For the most part, we will switch into System One, the automatic and often unconscious mode of decision making. If you are already hardwired to make a healthy choice, then that is no problem. If, however, your most common choices are less healthy, then it can be problematic.

The decisions don't stop there. With most offices having a snack dispenser, treats left on the side to celebrate a birthday or other landmark, and a local coffee shop selling food, calorie-rich goods are never far away.

Working from home presents different challenges. With the fridge and cupboards so close by, temptation is always within hand's reach.

Food and drink are hard to ignore. They surround us and are constantly advertised to us. Without a plan to circumnavigate all the temptation, the chances of avoiding it are slim.

Your eating habits are exactly that – habits. To improve them, the first step is to understand them. Awareness is the key to change. Once you have a better understanding of your routine, you can begin to add structure and plan ahead to reduce the number of food choices you need to make. This is arguably the most important phase of improving your eating habits.

Making changes to your diet without first taking time to find out what works well and what can be improved is like pinning a tail on a donkey blindfolded: you might hit the target, but you would have much better chance if you could see.

Get to know what you eat. Find out your calorie intake and get a better understanding of the food you most commonly consume and what things in your day impact your food choices.

By taking the time to find out this information, you'll be able to create an eating structure which works for your lifestyle, set yourself a calorie target which is aligned with your goals and improve your eating habits.

The first step is to track what you eat.

Food diary

It's incredible how many people dislike keeping a food diary. It's often seen as something that takes too much time and effort. In my experience, though, it's crucial for improving your diet and achieving your ideal body weight.

A study funded by the National Heart, Lung and Blood Institute at the National Institutes of Health, with more than 1,700 participants, found that keeping a food diary can double how much weight a person loses.[47] The knowledge of what you eat can make a massive impact on how you eat.

There are many reasons why keeping a diary of what you eat is essential:

1. You can find out precisely what you're eating (sounds obvious, but this is vital).

2. There's no better way to understand your eating habits, routines and trends.

3. If done honestly, a food diary alone can kick-start you into positive action.

4. You can view the percentages of carbohydrates, fat and protein you're eating.

5. You can see how many fruits and vegetables you consume.

6. You'll learn how many calories the food and drinks you consume contain (including alcohol).

7. It's a great tool to see how your eating habits are progressing.

8. It will help you realise what stops you from eating the right things or prevents you from eating altogether.

9. It begins a process of evaluation that will keep you consistent in years to come.

Though it's not something you need to do forever, keeping a food diary is essential at the start of your journey to better health. Over time, you'll understand the types of food you need to eat and how often to maintain your ideal weight. The simple truth is that you cannot master what you do not track.

When keeping a food diary, ensure that you include the following:

- The times you eat
- What meals you eat

- What snacks you eat

- What treats you eat

- What drinks you consume, including fizzy drinks and alcohol

I recommend keeping a food diary for the first three months, or until you've achieved your ideal body weight. After that point, I suggest keeping a journal every four to six weeks until you feel that eating a calorie-controlled diet has become second nature.

Be aware that many people track their calories inaccurately. One study found that when keeping a food diary, some participants underreported their calorie intake by as much as 1,000 calories per day.[48]

Even dietitians can get it wrong when reporting their calorie intake accurately, although to a lesser extent than the general public. Making a note of everything you eat, even down to the amount of oil and butter, will greatly improve the accuracy of your diary.[49]

Accuracy is one factor; consistency is another. It is common for people to track their food intake for a short period before stopping for two or three days, and then restarting again. Although you will still get a benefit from tracking for a couple of days, it will not give you a well-rounded view of your weekly eating habits. Consistently and accurately recording your food intake will give you an invaluable insight into your diet and calorie intake.

What you consume is just one factor when it comes to your eating habits. It's also important to find barriers that impact your ability to make healthier choices.

Your routine

While keeping your food diary, look for things that stop you from eating when and what you want to.

All the best-laid plans can be disrupted by outside circumstances, but we can plan ahead for things that commonly occur, such as:

- Meetings
- Travel
- Last-minute appointments
- People leaving treats around the office
- Work lunches
- Days out and events

Look at your diary to find trends in your routine so that you can make changes to your eating habits without disrupting your day. This is valuable information that will allow you to begin changing your eating habits to work better for you.

Also, look at what triggers a craving for a particular treat. For example, perhaps you have biscuits in your cupboard next to where you keep your teabags. The sight might trigger you to want a biscuit. Over time, you'll create an association between having a cup of tea and a biscuit. The first step is to remove the biscuits from your tea cupboard. Next, you'll need to have a replacement for the biscuit, such as a piece of fruit. This is just one example of how finding the initial trigger will allow you to make changes to your diet.

The goal is to make changes slowly, so as not to become overwhelmed.

There are many smartphone apps that you can use to track your meals. They make this process easy and, if you're someone who enjoys statistics, you'll find the data interesting.

Although this may seem like a lot of work, it will pay dividends in the long run. Your food choices will be healthier, and you'll make decisions around food efficiently. The aim is to create an environment that is conducive to making healthier choices.

EXERCISE

Begin keeping a food diary of everything that you eat. Make a note in your phone every time you consume food or drinks and put the time next to it. Also write down anything that triggers a craving for treats and at what time you had the craving. At the end of the day, add your meals, snacks and drinks into an online food tracker, so you can calculate your calorie intake.

At the end of the week, look at your notes and calorie intake. You will get a better understanding of your habits, what triggers you to make unhealthier choices and how many calories you consume each day.

Eating patterns

Instead of trying to find the perfect diet, create the ideal structure. Remember, you can stop dieting, but good habits will stick for life.

When you're busy or in a rush, bypass the need to make another choice by simplifying the process and customising your diet for your day. A Cornell study found that an average person makes more than 200 food choices in a day.[50] Limiting the options available will mean you're less likely to choose poorly.

At the start of the week, plan your meals, including snacks, based on when you usually want to eat. If your diary regularly changes, adjust your eating schedule accordingly. Again, this may seem like a lot of work, but it will save you time in the long run.

There are a number of ways that you can make this process easier:

- Do a weekly shop for everything you'll need. If you have time on a Sunday, prepare your meals for the rest of the week. If this isn't possible, ensure that you have dinner options that are quick and easy to prepare.

- Whenever you cook, make your meals in bulk and freeze them so you have options for when you don't have time to cook (or have the leftovers for lunch the next day).

- Prepare your breakfast in the evening so that you have a healthy option available in the morning. Preparation is key. It will save you time and mental energy.

- If you work in an office, prepare your lunch at home and take it with you. If that isn't possible, find three to five healthier go-to lunch options that you can grab when you're in a rush. Avoid the need to make a decision.

- If you often have work lunches or dinners, look at the menu before you go. This way, you can choose a healthy option beforehand, and you'll also have more time to speak with the people you're meeting with.

- Ensure your fridge is stocked with healthy options. Many people eat poorly when they come home from work hungry and don't have a quick and healthy option available.

- Remove all treat food from places in your cupboard that you regularly visit. Out of sight, out of mind.

- Have healthy snacks at hand during the day.

Life becomes easier when you prepare. You'll reduce the number of decisions you need to make, eat foods that are healthier and tastier, and have more time.

Key points

- The first step to improve your diet is to find out what you're eating. A food diary is an essential step to better eating habits.

- While tracking your food intake, look at what stops you from making the right food choices. Look for things that might trigger you to make poor choices and trends in your day that hinder your ability to eat when and what you want.

- With this information, begin to structure your meals around your week. It will save you time, reduce your chances of choosing food that isn't good for you and give you more freedom to enjoy treats without feeling guilt.

FREE GIFT

Download your free meal planner tool at
https://pathtopeakcondition.com/freegift

11
Energy Balance

If a household pet is overweight, the owner will likely first try to get it to move more and eat less, to lose the excess fat. They will follow this routine with an element of certainty that if they continue to exercise their pet and reduce the amount of food it consumes then it will end up losing weight. Although this may sound obvious, there are countless diets offering alternative approaches and there is no shortage of takers.

Whether your goal is to lose weight or gain muscle, you'll need to find the right energy balance.

The fundamental law of thermodynamics and numerous studies say that you'll begin to lose weight when you consume fewer calories than you expend.[51] On the flip side, if you want to gain weight and increase lean muscle, you'll need to be in a positive energy balance. There are many theories on dieting, but this one is hard to argue against – although many people try to. However, even though this is relatively straightforward in principle, it doesn't mean that finding the right balance is easy.

In this chapter we will look at how to find the right balance between calories in and calories out and some of the obstacles that can crop up along the way.

Energy in

Total daily energy expenditure

Multiple factors influence our total calorie intake. Everyone absorbs calories at different rates due to individual gut bacteria, so the same meal will be metabolised differently from person to person. This means that two people consuming the same meal will store a different number calories. Another factor is inaccuracies on food labels, calorie counters and restaurant menus. The Food and Drug Administration allows for inaccuracies of up to 20%.[52]

Calorie counting isn't an exact science, but it does give you a base to work from.

The first step is to set a calorie target based on your estimated total daily energy expenditure (TDEE). There are lots of apps and websites you can use to find this out. Once you have your TDEE, add either a surplus or a deficit, depending on your goal.

As a rough guide, if you want to lose weight and reduce body fat, I recommend a 10% to 20% calorie deficit. If you want to increase lean muscle, add a 5% to 15% surplus. This is dependent on your current body fat levels.

If you have a higher body fat percentage, you may want to start at a higher deficit; if you have lower body fat, your deficit should be lower. Ultimately, it's a process of testing and making adjustments to your calorie intake based on the results you see.

When assessing your calorie intake, look at it over a week instead of focusing solely on each day. Your intake will be higher on some days and lower on others. Most of the time, we consume more calories at the weekend than on weekdays because we have less structure at weekends. Look at the average to see if you've hit your target.

People often give themselves a hard time when they eat takeout or drink alcohol without knowing if it has impacted their average weekly calorie target over a week. But if the meal or drink was planned and you still hit your calorie target, there's no need to feel guilt.

This is one of the real benefits of tracking your calorie intake accurately and planning ahead. It allows more freedom to enjoy treats without worrying about it.

Be aware that staying in a calorie deficit for long periods can be stressful on the body. This means that cortisol levels increase, causing water retention.[53] The result is that you look bloated and feel soft to touch. Taking a break from dieting roughly every 12 weeks and increasing calorie consumption to a maintenance level will give the body a break and enable it to reduce cortisol levels.

Mindful Eating

Although calorie counting is extremely effective, it isn't for everyone. If you are someone who just can't get to grips with tracking your food, but still wants to get in good shape and improve your relationship with food, mindful eating is a good practice to follow.

Mindful eating involves purposeful focus on your food. This includes focusing on each mouthful, chewing your food properly and fully concentrating on its taste and texture. Mindful eating has been shown to reduce food cravings, emotional eating and body weight.[54]

We often eat without thinking. Use mindful eating to stop and assess hunger before eating. Ask yourself, 'Am I actually hungry?' Try to pinpoint why you are looking for something to snack on. Are you stressed, tired or emotional? Drink a glass of water before you make your decision. Often thirst is mistaken for hunger as the cue comes from the same part of our brain.

It is common to consume food while looking at our phones, working on a laptop or watching TV, but this can increase the amount we eat.[55] Switching off technology to fully focus on a meal makes us less likely to overeat.

I suggest practising mindful eating regardless of your goals, to improve your awareness of feelings of fullness and reduce your chance of overeating.

Energy out

Metabolic adaptation

Food was once hard to come by, so humans have evolved to store fat for periods of famine. Conserving energy was once essential for survival in winter months when food was sparse. When food was available, our ancestors would eat in abundance, search for energy-rich food and store excess calories as body fat. The extra energy would have allowed our ancestors to be more efficient in searching for food and shelter, competing for sexual partners, bearing children and avoiding predators.

Fast-forward to modern day: the most common jobs are sedentary and many of our food sources are calorie laden, but we still conserve excess energy as fat in preparation for the famine that never comes. This can make it difficult to lose weight and keep it off when we do.

When we lose weight, the body essentially defends the excess fat by slowing the rate at which we expend energy. This happens in several ways:

- Basal metabolic rate (BMR) declines. This is the minimum number of calories you need to keep your major organs operating, such as the heart, lungs and brain. When you weigh less, your body will need to expend fewer calories to keep you functioning. *BMR accounts for 60% to 80% of TDEE.*

- Exercise activity thermogenesis (EAT) declines. This is how many calories your body uses during dedicated exercise. When you eat less, you have less energy to exercise, increasing the chances of missing sessions or not training as vigorously when you do. You're therefore likely to burn fewer calories through activity. You'll also expend less energy when you do exercise because it doesn't require as many calories to move a smaller body around. *EAT accounts for 10% of TDEE.*

- Non-exercise activity thermogenesis (NEAT) declines. This is how many calories you use when moving around (fidgeting, standing and walking).

Less food means less energy, so you're likely to naturally move less, and when you do, you'll burn fewer calories due to being lighter. *NEAT makes up 10% to 20% of TDEE.*

- Thermic effect of food (TEF) declines. This is how many calories your body uses to digest food. When you eat less, you burn fewer calories. Digestion will also slow down so that your body can absorb as many nutrients as possible, meaning you store more of the calories that you eat. *TEF accounts for 10% of the TDEE.*

Although when we lose weight, our metabolic rate is expected to reduce in tandem because of the reasons above, there can be excessive reduction from severe calorie restriction which exceeds the expected change – eg you lose 10% body weight and your metabolic rate declines by 15%. This is called metabolic adaptation, also known as adaptive thermogenesis. The severity and longevity of this response varies from study to study.

Although the reasons for metabolic adaptation are not fully understood and the effects can vary from person to person, there are strategies to counter the effects of a slower metabolism and continue to lose weight.

Lean muscle

Maintaining lean muscle mass is one of the most important factors to achieve sustainable weight loss. Lean

127

muscle is metabolically more active than fat tissue so burns more calories. It's estimated that every half a kilogram of muscle burns six calories per day at rest. This is three times as many calories as half a kilogram of fat. For example, if someone lost 4.5 kg of fat and gained 4.5 kg of lean muscle, they would burn 40 more calories per day.[56] This is just one example of how you can train your body to burn calories more efficiently.

The most effective way to increase lean muscle is to take part in progressive resistance training, which we discussed in strength. During exercise we cause muscle damage; in the recovery phase, cells produce protein to repair the damaged muscle. This process is called protein synthesis.

Think of resistance training as the bulldozer breaking down a wall, protein as the bricks needed to rebuild it and protein synthesis as the builder repairing the damage. This process requires a lot of energy and raises your metabolism.

A reduction in muscle mass is one of the reasons that crash dieting can be an ineffective way to maintain weight loss. Too high a calorie deficit can result in muscle loss, which can slow the metabolic rate, making it harder to keep the weight off when the weight loss goal is achieved.[57] Reducing calorie intake too drastically can also impact energy levels and make it harder to reach the intensity needed when working out to maintain or increase lean muscle. It is a fine balancing act when in a calorie deficit.

It's essential to continue resistance training to preserve lean muscle all the way through life. This will aid weight management and overall health.

Protein

One aspect of weight loss that is almost universally accepted is that adequate protein intake is essential.

Unlike carbohydrates and fat, protein cannot be stored in high quantities – the body either breaks it down into amino acids and transports it to various part of the body to repair and build things, such as muscle, or excretes it.

To maintain or increase muscle, the body must have a net positive protein balance. This means that you need to keep replenishing stores by consuming enough protein daily. The amount of protein needed depends on several factors, including age, physical activity and the amount of lean muscle mass, but a good starting point is 1.6 g per kilogram of body weight.[58] If you have a lower body fat percentage, I recommend a slightly higher protein intake; if your body fat percentage is higher, your intake can be slightly lower.

Another positive of consuming adequate protein: protein requires more energy to digest than carbohydrates and fat, so TEF will increase when you eat it. Research shows that 20–30% of the total calories in protein are used to digest it. Carbohydrates use 5–10% and fats 0–3%.[59]

Be aware that entering a calorie deficit can cause a decrease in protein synthesis, which, as discussed, is the process in which cells make proteins.[60]

Spreading your protein intake over three to five meals will help keep your protein synthesis level elevated, aiding muscle growth and recovery. Don't overthink this; simply being in a calorie deficit is enough at the beginning. As we have seen, when we lose weight NEAT declines, so we expend less energy. Therefore it is essential to create a strategy to stay active.

NEAT

A strategy often overlooked when discussing the energy–balance equation is simply moving more.

A study by the National Weight Control Registry, which is the biggest of its kind, tracked 10,000 people who lost a significant amount of weight and kept it off. The researchers looked at common habits that enabled each individual to be successful when so many others struggled to maintain their weight loss. Almost every participant increased their physical activity, and walking was the most common form of exercise.[61] Other studies have supported the importance of remaining active for weight management.[62]

Increasing your daily step count is vital. I highly recommend monitoring it. Wearing a smartwatch is shown to increase daily step count by 27%. Smartphones can also track your step count but aren't as accurate.[63]

As a guideline – a person with a step count below 5,000 per day would be considered sedentary and one with 10,000 would be considered active. It's not uncommon for people who spend most of the day seated to have step counts in the low thousands. This is why tracking your step count is crucial. Awareness is the key to change. Ten thousand steps daily is an excellent target to aim for and equates to roughly 7.5 km, depending on your stride length.[64]

Here's some context around how an increased step count can accumulate. Taking an extra 2,000 steps each day equates to:

- 1.5 km per day
- 10.5 km per week
- 45 km per month
- 547.5 km per year

Someone of average height who weighed 73 kg would burn roughly 40 calories per 1,000 steps over a year – an extra 29,200 calories burned, or 4.5 kg of weight.

When you put an extra 2000 steps per day into this context, you can see the power of the daily walk.

Another way to increase your step count is to take the stairs instead of the lift. Do it each time you come in or out of work, and the steps will quickly accumulate. Also, avoid standing on escalators whenever possible.

It's faster and much healthier. I always find it strange that after a full day of sitting at a desk, people will stand on the escalator and then fight for a seat on the train.

When travelling to and from work, get off a stop early and walk the rest of the way. Leave your car at home and walk to the shops when possible. Instead of emailing or calling a colleague, walk over and speak to them. Or email them and then walk over. Ask for an adjustable desk at work so that you can move between standing and sitting at regular intervals. If you work from home and don't have an adjustable desk, move from kneeling to seated. This will help you avoid spending too long in the same position.

The energy–balance equation is key to achieving a healthy body weight.

Key points

- To lose weight, we need to be in a calorie deficit by consuming fewer calories than we expend. Calorie counting isn't an exact science but gives you a base to work from. You can then set a target and begin adapting based on the results you see.

- As you lose weight, the body reduces its metabolic rate in a process called metabolic adaptation. At this point, it's important to reduce calorie intake.

- You can reduce the impact of metabolic adaptation by performing resistance training and increasing protein intake to preserve lean muscle while tracking your step count to ensure you remain active.

12
80/20

No food is inherently bad for us. It is the quantity of certain types of food that can be.

Finding balance in your diet is a crucial element of sustainable eating habits. There are diets which pre-scribe only eating like a hunter-gatherer and others that suggest removing a macronutrient such as fat or carbohydrates. There are shake diets, cabbage soup diets, no sugar diets – and the list goes on.

The problem with each of these diets is that they seem to forget that eating different types of food is one of life's pleasures. Sweets, pastries and chocolate taste good, but if you eat them all the time the pleasure begins to subside. The same is true of only eating takeaways.

If I go for a few days without eating any fruit or vegetables I start to crave them and the satisfied feeling that comes with consuming nutrient-dense food. Taking a balanced approach is essential.

Too much highly processed food is bad for us, but removing it completely is unsustainable for most of us. We will look at how to find the right balance, but first, we'll discuss processed food.

Processed food

To achieve and maintain your ideal weight, you will need to achieve energy balance. You can lose weight by eating a highly processed diet as long as you are in a calorie deficit, but not only is it not a healthy way to eat, it will make the process much harder.

In one study, twenty participants were allowed to eat an uncontrolled amount of processed food over two weeks, followed by two more weeks in the same conditions but this time eating unprocessed food. Not surprisingly, the participants gained weight when eating processed food and lost weight when eating unprocessed food. They ate 508 more calories per day in the first two weeks.[65]

As discussed, highly processed food is pleasurable and can be addictive. Also, it's often low in nutrients and won't leave us satisfied. The result is that we'll keep eating, searching for the high that comes from consuming this type of food.

Eating less processed food and a diet high in real, whole food will help you avoid this scenario, and eating foods that have a low calorie density will allow you to eat more and reduce cravings while still cutting back on calories.

Real, whole food

I often get asked which type of food is best for losing or maintaining weight, and my answer is always the same: eat real, whole food whenever possible – lots of fruits and vegetables, nuts and seeds, legumes and beans, whole grains, herbs and spices, and healthy fats (eg olive oil and oily fish). Limit processed foods and sugars from sources such as high-fructose corn syrup.

My recommendation is similar to a traditional Mediterranean diet. According to the Harvard School of Public Health, 'Together with regular physical activity and not smoking... over 80% of coronary heart disease, 70% of stroke, and 90% of type 2 diabetes can be avoided by healthy food choices that are consistent with the traditional Mediterranean diet.'[66] And a study published in *The New England Journal of Medicine* showed that the traditional Mediterranean diet is associated with a reduction in total mortality.[67]

Though the Mediterranean diet has many health benefits, the term still suggests it's 'a diet' instead of 'your diet'. Really, it's just a way of eating. This is why I tell people to eat whole, real food.

There is no ideal macronutrient split between protein, fat and carbohydrates in a whole, real-food diet.[68] As we have discussed, maintaining a relatively high protein intake is important for maintaining and building lean muscle. This has many benefits, from weight management to boosting the immune system.

Consuming adequate healthy fats is essential for optimal health, but be aware that they are also higher in calories than carbohydrates and protein. There are four calories per gram of protein and carbohydrate, but nine calories per gram of fat.[69] This means you'll be able to eat substantially less healthy fat than fibrous carbohydrates and proteins.

If you are in a calorie deficit, I recommend a higher consumption of food with a low calorie density. One of the main reasons is that you will simply be able to consume more food. Hunger is one of the toughest parts of being in a calorie deficit. Filling your plate with low-calorie-dense food will leave you feeling fuller for longer.

Calorie density relates to number of calories in food compared to the volume or weight. Generally, foods that are high in fibre and water have a low calorie density. Food with a high water content will expand the stomach, which means you'll feel fuller for longer. One of the reasons that dietary fibre will leave you feeling fuller is because it includes the parts of plant foods your body can't digest or absorb. This means that you'll excrete most of what you eat. This is important when you're trying to lose weight or maintain your ideal weight.

Filling your plate with more leafy vegetables while reducing rice or pasta is a great way to increase satiety and reduce calories. Add a healthy serving of fats and a generous serving of protein and you will have a highly nutritious and calorie-controlled meal.

When you eat whole, real food, you'll be able to eat more while consuming fewer calories, compared to a diet with lots of highly processed food. Plus, real, whole food is nutrient dense compared to processed food, which often has little nutritional value.

That is not to say that processed food is inherently bad. It is the volume and frequency of consumption that can be. This is where 80/20 split can be so beneficial. It allows for treats but on your terms, as part of a well-rounded diet.

Finding balance

It's nigh on impossible to eat well all the time, and to be frank, who would want to? Life is to be enjoyed, and the odd treat is undoubtedly one of life's pleasures.

I advise living by the 80/20 rule. Simply eat real, whole foods 80% of the time and treat yourself for the remaining 20%. If you're in a calorie deficit, an 80/20 split will make the process much easier to sustain. Reducing calories is tough at times, so adding treats into your week is critical to ensure that you can reward your effort and feel 'normal'. You may be tempted to stop all treat foods, but this approach rarely works. It can seem like a long, uphill struggle if you never have any downtime.

There are many times where what we eat is out of our control, or our options are reduced, such as at work events, dinner parties or when travelling, so be sure to save some of your 20% for moments like these – factor them into your weekly plan.

Depending on your current eating habits, it may take time to get to an 80/20 split. Gradually change the percentages until you get to this point.

The 80/20 rule comes with a warning: be aware that treat foods are generally much more energy-dense than real, whole foods, so this doesn't mean 20% of your meals but 20% of your overall calorie intake – and yes, the 20% includes alcohol consumption.

The 80/20 rule is the optimal ratio for a healthy and sustainable diet, but the food we consume is just half of the story. Drinking enough water plays an important role in satiety, energy and overall health.

EXERCISE

What is your current split between real, whole foods and treats?

Look at how you can begin improving the ratio by looking first at your breakfast, then lunch and finally dinner.

Water

The average human body is made up of roughly 60% water. If you've lost even 1% or 2% of that water, you'll start to experience fatigue, reduced endurance, concentration and coordination, and headaches.[70]

Water helps break down food, aid nutrient consumption and boost blood circulation. Dehydration can make you feel hungry when, in fact, you're simply thirsty. You may think you need food or have low blood sugar when you need a glass of water.

Make sure you're fully hydrated before each meal. Drinking 16 oz of water half an hour before you eat has been shown to speed up fat loss in obese adults.[71] As mentioned, this works because you feel full when your stomach is stretched. Drinking water before a meal essentially tricks hunger sensors into thinking you're full.

There are ways to spot dehydration:

- Dry mouth and lips

- Dark urine (aim for it to be light yellow or clear)

- Low energy levels

- Slight headache

Always keep a BPA-free bottle of water by you and sip from it regularly throughout the day. This will give you a better idea of how much you're drinking each day. If you find it hard to drink plain water, flavour it with a slice or two of cucumber or a sprig of mint – you might be surprised by how much you can drink.

The final piece of the puzzle

Creating structure in your eating habits so they match your lifestyle, finding the right energy balance to achieve your aesthetic goals and sticking to the 80/20 rule are the most sustainable and enjoyable ways to approach your diet. Getting to this stage takes time and consistency, but before long, it will become an ingrained behaviour and a lifestyle choice.

We've now looked at both exercise and diet. The final piece of the puzzle is recovery.

Recovery is the missing link for many busy people. We live in a society where a 'sleep less and work more' philosophy is often endorsed, but too much work without adequate recovery will ultimately lead to a declining performance.

Achieving this balance is harder than ever, but it's possible, and when you get it right, every area of life improves.

Key points

- Trying to cut out all processed food is unsustainable. Find a balance by consuming roughly 80% of your calories from whole, real food and saving 20% for treats.

- Eating a diet of whole, real food has many health benefits and will enable you to eat more while consuming fewer calories compared to eating a diet of highly processed food.

- Dehydration can lead to fatigue and reduced concentration and coordination. It may also create the sensation of hunger. Try to keep a bottle of water nearby and drink from it regularly throughout the day.

FREE GIFT

You can download your free weight-loss manual at www.pathtopeakcondition.com/freegift

13
Introduction To Recovery

Stress is often discussed in a negative context, but it's essential and can elevate our performance. Stress itself isn't the problem – it's the quantity and intensity of it that can be. The antidote to stress is recovery. It is the counterbalance that enables you to harness the positive effects of stress.

You will go through periods of high stress. They are necessary to force adaptation and improve in all areas of life. When you find the right balance between stress and recovery, you experience eustress – the positive form of stress.

About twenty years after the release of *The Stress of Life*, Hans Selye introduced a theory suggesting that stress can be both positive and negative. These two forms of stress are called 'eustress' and 'distress'. Eustress is positive; it helps us to stay motivated, driven and improves performance. Distress, on the other hand, is negative; it leads to overwhelm, increases anxiety and reduces performance.[72]

Take the scenario of working on a big project. You're excited about the new task. You wake up nervous but focused on working hard to achieve the desired outcome. At the start, you're able to handle the volume of work. You enjoy the process and feel in control, and the project seems to be progressing nicely.

Suddenly, there's a cut to the budget, you lose a few team members and your workload increases. You begin to struggle and fall behind schedule. Your days become longer, you eat whenever possible and have fewer breaks, and the quality of your work begins to decline.

After sustaining this intensity for a while, you succumb to the pressure, and everything begins to fall apart. The project is no longer fun or rewarding; instead, it's overwhelming, and you feel unable to cope.

This is an example of moving from eustress to distress.

In the beginning, you're excited. Your stress energises and motivates you, and you feel in control of the situation. As the volume of work increases, though, you fall out of routine and begin to lose control. This triggers anxiety, and your performance begins to decline.

Studies show that the more a person feels in control of a situation, the less likely they are to feel distress. This is especially true in a work environment.[73]

We often feel in control when we have time for ourselves and follow a structured routine. Over the years, I've spoken to countless people who struggle to find time for themselves. Simple tasks such as going for a walk, taking time for lunch or scheduling a workout are no longer possible. At this point, they live in a state of 'fight or flight' for much of the day. If this sounds familiar, you need to break the cycle.

The way you structure your day will have a big impact on whether you experience eustress or distress. If you want to progress toward your goals and perform at your best, it is essential to create a balanced lifestyle which stimulates eustress.

Your ability to manage stress is strongly influenced by three factors:

- **Morning routine:** The way you begin your day has a big impact on how you feel throughout it. Following a structured morning routine will ensure you start the day in a calm and focused manner.

- **Reset periods:** Finding moments in your day to get some downtime will enable you to reset and refocus on the next task at hand.

- **Pre-bed ritual:** Your routine leading up to bedtime will greatly impact your quality of sleep and how you feel the following day.

The way you begin the day has a massive impact on how you feel for the rest of it. This is what we'll look at first.

14
Morning Routine

I used to wake up in a bad mood. I'd be annoyed if someone simply spoke to me, and the conversation in my head would go something like this: 'Why are you talking to me? Do you not know the time?'

This was obviously not a good way to begin the day – for me or anyone who was unfortunate enough to be around me. I knew things had to change, so I started to research ways to improve my mindset first thing.

I looked at how to improve my sleep quality so that I'd wake up feeling fresh and more awake, and at what I could do in the morning so that I got off to a flying start. What I discovered transformed my whole day.

Now, I get up at 5am each day. Try to get up at least 1 hour before anyone else in your household. After other people in your house wake up and you get into the routine of your day, you lose a certain amount of control. Anything can happen, but that first hour, before other people are around – that's yours.

Now, my routine is structured like a military operation, with everything in its place so that I can glide through my morning and get off to the best possible start. When my alarm goes off, I make sure that I win the first challenge, which is to get out of bed straight away.

My routine has become habitual, and I've achieved my desired result: I'm happy as soon as I wake in the morning and look forward to the next day each evening before bed. A few simple changes have truly changed my world and allowed me to be happier and more focused throughout my day, and face the challenges that it brings.

I've passed this routine on to countless clients, and they too have benefited from this positive start to the day.

The routine you develop will be personal. Mine includes kissing my partner, looking in on my children and stroking my dog, Arnie. Whatever else you include in your morning routine, there are three things I recommend doing:

1. Meditate

2. Warm up for the day

3. Appreciate what you have

Meditate

It's easy to check your phone first thing and instantly switch on to the demands of the day. What you see can impact your mindset. Try to avoid looking at any messages for the first hour and meditate instead.

Meditation allows me to chart my mental state first thing. If I've had a bad sleep or woken up with things on my mind, it will take longer to calm my mind. This signals to me that I might be in a heightened state of stress and is a warning that I could react too fast in situations and not come across the way I want to.

If I have a meeting in the morning, I'll make sure that I mentally prepare. This means considering how I want to be seen in that environment. I'll be more likely to carry baggage into the meeting if I'm not in a calm state. Acting out of character never feels good and only adds to internal stress. Use meditation as your assessment tool each morning.

It will bring you a sense of calm and set you up for any challenges ahead. It will also allow you to stay focused on a given task – to get into a flow state, or 'in the zone'. When you're in a flow state, you're absorbed in what you're doing, meaning that the quality of your output and your productivity will likely be improved.

Top poker players win because of their ability to focus and read their opponents' body language. They see signs that indicate either a good or bad hand. This unwavering concentration is the difference between winning a large sum of money or losing one. If they didn't hone their mental skills, they'd be relying much more on luck.

Improved focus also allows us to see and hear more in situations such as important meetings and conversations. When you give someone your full attention, you'll pick up body-language cues and gain a better understanding of what's needed.

Meditation can be viewed as a mental workout. It will increase your ability to fully focus for longer periods, and it will help you make decisions from a calmer state of mind. You'll be able to mentally step back from a situation and react in a controlled and thoughtful manner – to *review situations instead of simply reacting to them.*

Meditation is a skill, an addition to your artillery. It has been used for generations to improve mental performance, and you can use it too.

If you're new to meditation, begin with just a few minutes – trying to stay focused for too long at the start can be stressful. Find a quiet space away from distractions. Then get into a comfortable sitting position (avoid lying down, as it's easy to fall back to sleep), close your eyes and start to concentrate on your breath. Thoughts will enter your mind, and that's fine; just accept them before refocusing on your breathing. Try to be happy in this moment, even if you're not in a particularly good mood. A simple trick is to smile. Smiling can release your mood-boosting neurotransmitters, such as dopamine and serotonin, making you feel happier.

Many people are put off by meditation because they believe that they should be able to clear their mind of all thoughts, but this is simply not true. Thoughts will come in and out of your mind, and you'll get better at controlling them. There's a reason people say they 'practise meditation'. Expect it to take time before you're comfortable with the process. You may wish to try one of the many meditation apps to get started.

When I decided to meditate, I knew that I'd need structure to stay consistent. Since I wanted to meditate first thing, I paired it with my morning coffee. When I wake up, I head downstairs and switch on my coffee maker. This works as a trigger to go and meditate. I go to the same area in my house, sit in the same spot and follow the same process. Once I've finished meditating, I make my coffee, which also acts as a reward.

As I added more things to my morning routine, I used old habits as triggers to form the new ones. You can do this with any habit you want to add to your routine. Find a current habit and place the new practice you wish to ingrain next to it.

Warm up for the day

Just as you warm up to work out, warm up for your day. You're likely going to be in the same position for long periods, so you need to move your joints through their full range of motion. As discussed in Chapter 7, this involves doing joint rotations.

Moving mindfully is also a form of meditation and will give you better awareness of your body. We're often so consumed with technology and the demands of daily life that we forget how to connect with our body. Taking time first thing in the morning to feel how each joint is moving will highlight areas that are uncomfortable and give you a better understanding of how you move.

Meditation and movement will increase your ability to get into the flow state, enabling you to focus your attention more intently on a given task during the day.

Appreciate what you have

I believe that being happy can take work and that life is all about perception. What may annoy you may not annoy others, and vice versa.

Taking a few minutes each morning to think about the good things in your life – and there will be plenty – will set you up for a positive day. Thinking about what you have and being thankful for it will place you in a happier, more relaxed state. The happier you are, the healthier you are.

When you have a negative start to the day, more negative things seem to creep in. Don't allow this to happen to you. Being grateful is one of the best ways to stay positive.

It's easy to forget all the good things we have in life as we strive for the next achievement. The highs that come with buying a new item or achieving a new milestone are short-lived before normality returns. This is called the hedonic treadmill.

The hedonic treadmill is a theory that people have a set level of happiness that they will return to, even after experiencing positive or negative events. If you won the lottery, the high of this experience would pass, only to be replaced by the same worries and problems that once concerned you. Conversely, if you lost a limb, you'd soon adapt to this new reality.

Having gratitude opens you up to enjoy the day just for being another day.

Taking a few moments each morning to consider all the positive things in your life will enrich your day and start you off on a high. Many of the world's most successful people credit gratitude as one of the keys to their success. If it benefits them, it may well help you too.

The way you begin the day will have a profound impact on the rest of it. Prioritise your first hour so that you get off to the best possible start.

Once you have a structured morning routine, the next step is to focus on adding moments of mental down-time to your day.

EXERCISE

Consider how you start your morning and think about how you can get off to the best possible start.

Which of the three suggestions above could you add into your morning routine?

Key points

- The way you begin the day will have a big impact on how you feel during it. Following a structured morning routine will increase your chances of starting on the right foot.

- Meditation has many mental and physical benefits. Adding it into your morning will leave you feeling calmer and more focused for the upcoming day. Start with just a few minutes and increase the duration gradually.

- Adding a movement practice to your morning routine will add another layer of mindfulness to your day. Follow it with some gratitude, so that you begin on a positive note.

15
Reset Periods

Finding times to rest and reset in a busy day is crucial. Even the briefest moment to switch down gears can remove us from a state of fight, flight or freeze and bring calm. If you are used to being busy, you will likely have become habitually busy, and even when there are moments to relax, it can be difficult to do so.

Think of being in a one-to-one client meeting. Your client excuses themselves and goes to the bathroom. You instantly check your phone and begin looking at and replying to emails. As your client returns, you quickly finish off replying to one last message and switch back to your meeting.

Instead of scanning the room and giving your brain a crucial moment of mental downtime, you have spent the time focused on another task. This is how many people spend much of their day: moving from one task to the next, one stressor to another, never giving themselves a breather.

When a day is in full flow it can feel like there is no time, but there is often more than we believe. It is simply about planning downtime just as you do meetings and work commitments and creating a habit of switching off when there is an opportunity to do so.

In this chapter, we will look at strategies that I use in my life and have passed on to clients that allow for brief and important moments of downtime, to rest and reset.

Break the smartphone habit

From first thing in the morning until last thing at night, we're switched on. Many people check their phones out of habit, even when they haven't been triggered by an alert. Technology is essentially training us to self-interrupt. We search for the dopamine release that comes with a new message, with a new email or with a 'like' or comment on our social media pages. This quick hit of the reward hormone is short-lived, leaving us waiting for the next fix.

Families check their phones at the dinner table instead of talking and enjoying their meal. Shoppers get in line and instantly pull out their phones. People walk down the street with their eyes glued to their phones and their ears plugged with earphones, taking in little notice of their surroundings.

According to research from RescueTime, an app created to monitor phone use, on average, people spend 3 hours and 15 minutes on their phones each day and check them fifty-eight times.[74]

If we don't give ourselves mental downtime, our nervous system never shuts down. We're in a constant state of fight or flight, always switched on, feeling wired and tired much of the time. We turn off the TV when we leave the room, and we let our computer reboot, but we often don't allow our brains to do the same.

Finding ways to break the habit of checking our phone is becoming ever more important. Here are a few tips that have allowed me to reduce my screen time:

- Remove any notifications that aren't essential, such as app notifications, so you aren't prompted to look at your phone.

- Aim to put your phone in another room 90 minutes before you sleep and collect it 1 hour after you wake up. Invest in an old-fashioned alarm clock instead of using your phone. This will allow you to have an extended period without your phone and reduce the chance that you'll check it before bed or when you wake up.

- Place your phone in another room while relaxing.
- Assign dedicated time to check messages, emails and social media.
- Avoid looking at your phone while eating and concentrate fully on your food. This will allow you mental downtime and will also help you eat mindfully.

As with any habit, you'll need to set up a system to break it.

Finding moments to switch off during the day is crucial to your well-being and performance. There are many tactics you can use to reset in a busy schedule, starting with finding a space where you won't be interrupted.

Mental downtime

At the start of my career, I was fortunate to land a coaching role within a blue-chip company. I quickly built up a good client base, and before long, I was busy with clients for much of the day, with little time for recovery.

Coaching people for long periods can take up a lot of mental energy, and I pushed myself hard. For the short breaks that I did have, I'd try to avoid conversation. The one place of solitude I could find was in the toilets, so that's where I'd go, even if I wasn't in need. It became my regular haunt, the place where I'd remove myself from any mental stimulation. I'd just sit there and shut my eyes for a few glorious moments. This respite was my saviour. It allowed me to continue working with many clients and maintain a high quality of work. The fact that I was fit and ate a well-rounded diet also helped me manage this intense workload.

I thought my toilet hideout was unusual, but I've since learned from clients and friends in the business world that this isn't uncommon. Lots of people find a few moments in the smallest room to get away from the stress of work and the demands others would place on them. Those four walls offer solace from others who want their time and is sometimes the only chance they have to take deep breaths and relax. I'm sure that not many people would talk about it, let alone admit to it for a book, but it does happen – and regularly.

Physiologically, you may be in a state of fight or flight for most of your day, so it makes sense that the instinct is to find a place of safety. The problem is that even in a toilet cubicle, you're not alone. Smartphones can follow you into this safe zone, and if you're not careful, instead of unwinding, you'll be checking emails. Even when working from home, it is not unusual to spend much of the day on video calls with few breaks.

It's essential to take moments of mental downtime. Wherever you choose to do so, make sure you avoid any mental stimulation. Just close your eyes and breathe deeply, even if you have only a couple of minutes.

Breathe deeply

Even the briefest moment is an opportunity to take a deep breath – and the benefits are wide reaching.

Deep breathing relieves stress because it signals to the brain to calm down. The brain then relays that message to the body, and you relax. Your blood pressure and heart rate will decrease, and you enter a calmer state.[75]

Although finding downtime in your day can be difficult, remember that you need only need a couple of minutes.

A study led by Michael Melnychuk, a researcher at the Trinity College Institute of Neuroscience in Dublin, Ireland, revealed that noradrenaline, a stress hormone, changed a region in the brain called the locus coeruleus, which is believed to have a role in attention control. The researchers found that 'our attention is influenced by our breath and that it rises and falls with the cycle of respiration. It is possible that by focusing on and regulating your breathing you can optimise your attention level and likewise, by focusing on your attention level, your breathing becomes more synchronised'.[76] Deep breathing leaves us calmer and more focused.

Your diaphragm plays a significant role in breathing by increasing the volume of your thorax and inflating your lungs. This helps you to breathe deeper and longer. Your diaphragm is like any other muscle: if you don't regularly use it, it will become weaker, reducing your capacity to consume oxygen. When you practise deep breathing, you strengthen your diaphragm. This allows you to oxygenate your blood more efficiently.[77]

Here's a simple technique. Place your hand on your belly before breathing in deeply through your nose for 4 seconds. Let your belly expand and your ribs separate as you hold the breath for 1 second. Then slowly breathe out through pursed lips – as if you were blowing a whistle – for 8 seconds, until you have no more air in your lungs and your ribcage has pulled towards your belly button.

I like to imagine my nose being on my belly button and each breath inflating my stomach. I focus entirely on each breath as it enters and leaves my body. It's essential to breathe in through your nose – it takes longer to fill your diaphragm this way, so your lungs can extract more oxygen.

This is unbelievably relaxing, and only one or two deep breaths are needed to be effective.

Walk

While at a retreat in Sri Lanka with my partner, I spent some time with a Buddhist monk called Guru Garvin. At the age of eighty-two, Guru Garvin could bend his body into positions that most people achieve only when they're children. He looked as if he were always in a trance. As he spoke, his eyes would roll to the back of his head.

Each day, we'd sit on the concrete temple floor practising meditation before talking. Garvin told me he'd meditated every day since he was ten years old and often had out-of-body experiences where he could look down on himself from above.

We spoke about health and well-being and the differences between his life and mine, which were worlds apart. Garvin lived a calm life, whereas mine is busy. He explained that finding moments to switch off was key to living a long and fulfilled life and that any situation was an opportunity for mindfulness.

One day, he taught me about walking meditation. 'When you walk,' he said, 'bring your attention to the present moment. Think about each step, the movement of your legs and your feet making contact with the ground or floor. Take in the sounds around you. Focus your attention on whatever your eyes take in. Each time you practise, focus your attention for slightly longer.'

Although being in the present can be difficult, the more we practise doing so, the better we become at it. This is where walking can be so beneficial. It allows us to downshift in a fast-paced world.

I use what I call '10 Minute Matters' to take short exercise breaks away from my desk to reset and refocus. At the start of your week, schedule 10 minutes for walking each day into your diary. For these 10 minutes, leave your phone at home or in the office. This will allow you to get some fresh air without any interruptions.

It may feel uncomfortable not having your phone at first. Remember, creating a new habit takes time. You'll get used to it soon enough. Walk on your own or with a friend or colleague; the only proviso is to avoid talking about work or any other problems – this is a time to laugh, smile and switch off from the demands of your day.

A study by Draugiem Group, which tracked the work habits of its employees, found that a work-to-rest ratio of 52 minutes of work followed by 17 minutes of rest was ideal for focus and productivity. The key was that when the most productive employees returned to work after their break, they focused solely on the task at hand, ignoring any distractions, including checking emails and social media accounts.[78]

This working method negates cognitive boredom, often brought on by doing the same task for long periods. It allows your brain to naturally ebb and flow. Taking a short break to go out for a walk will make you more productive on your return.

You can also use the benefit of walking when in meetings. I know a senior leader who often takes walking meetings. She believes it increases creativity, and there's evidence to back up her theory. A study at Stanford University compared walking to sitting in terms of how they affected creativity. They found that walking increased creative output by 60%.[79] If you're on a call, try to walk around instead of sitting.

A daily walk is a primary resource to unwind and refocus, and it's vital to maintain optimal mental and physical health.

If possible, try to take your walk during daylight hours. One in five people in the UK is low in vitamin D.[80] Vitamin D is produced naturally by the body when it's directly exposed to sunlight.

Vitamin D plays an essential role in mood regulation.[81] It also promotes healthy bones and teeth by increasing absorption of calcium, among many other health benefits.

Although there's nothing better than getting vitamin D through sunlight, this can sometimes be difficult, so make sure you're getting it through other sources as well, such as certain foods and supplements.

EXERCISE

Look at your diary and schedule in a 10-minute break to take a walk each day.

Those 10 minutes will become an integral part of your recovery strategy.

Find a hobby

Taking moments of downtime during your workday is crucial, but it's also important to make time in your private life to fully de-stress for the sake of your mental health.

My mother, who has had severe depression, credits her time spent alone painting as a key to her remarkable recovery. She says, 'Painting allows me to completely cut off from the outside world and fully focus my attention. I enter a complete state of flow, and for those moments I have no awareness of the outside world.'

My mum isn't alone in her belief that a focused hobby is important for mental well-being. Winston Churchill once said, 'Painting is complete as a distraction. I know of nothing which, without exhausting the body, more entirely absorbs the mind.'[82]

Finding ways to switch off from the outside world will improve your focus and calm your mind. The ability to tune out the world's noise and concentrate on one task that you enjoy might be pivotal in maintaining good mental health.

My mum is proof.

Key points

- Creating strategies to switch off during the day is fundamental to maintain high performance. Because of our technology, we're more switched on than ever before. Take time away from your screens so your brain can enjoy some important downtime.

- Throughout your day, take a few deep breaths without any outside interruptions. This will improve your focus and leave you feeling calmer. A great way to downshift is to go for a mindful walk daily. Even a 10-minute walk will have a big impact on how you feel.

- A relaxing hobby which enables you to completely remove yourself from the demands of a busy day will help you rest and reset.

16
Pre-bed Ritual

After my son was born, my partner and I experienced what new parents throughout the world go through: sleepless nights. There's no way to prepare for the challenges a newborn brings. I like to describe it as being put into a tumble dryer before someone presses 'fast spin'. It's a fantastic experience but highly challenging. Your regular routine suddenly changes, as you must dedicate your time to looking after a totally reliant human being.

Not only does the day change, the night does too. For me, good-quality sleep soon became a distant memory. Before long, a level of sleep deprivation kicked in that I never knew was possible. Although at the time I believed that I was functioning well, I was nowhere near my best. I was working the same hours but getting less done. I couldn't concentrate as I'd once been able to, I had less drive and I procrastinated.

Numerous studies have shown the impact of a poor night's sleep on focus, drive and even memory consolidation.[83] Sleep is also the primary way we 'empty the bucket of water'. Without a good night's sleep, we wake up with the bucket half full, so our tolerance to the day's stressors will be lower.

As well as being less productive, I struggled to work out. Not only did I have less energy, but I also lacked motivation to exercise. I decreased the intensity of my sessions as I simply couldn't elevate my performance. My goal became maintenance instead of progress. Instead of giving it my all, I simply 'got through' each workout.

This shouldn't have come as a surprise.

Sleep and exercise

Sleep plays a vital role in creating testosterone and growth hormones – hormones that boost performance and increase lean muscle. A poor night's sleep reduces the production of testosterone and growth hormones, increases recovery time and can impact lean muscle growth.

Suboptimal sleep also reduces the body's ability to replenish muscle glycogen, which is the main form of energy we use during exercise. Less glycogen means reduced total work capacity and muscle function. Without deep sleep, the mobilisation of free fatty acids, which help combat muscle breakdown caused by working out, and protein synthesis decline.

Poor sleep can impact your CNS's ability to recuperate, and your fitness may suffer. The CNS is responsible for pain response, muscle contractions and reaction time. This means you'll become slower, weaker and maybe even less coordinated in your workouts. A review in *Sports Medicine* showed that a bad night's sleep could make a workout feel harder and lead to quicker fatigue.[84]

It's no wonder my exercise routine was impacted, and it wasn't the only thing that was affected – my diet also suffered. The change in my routine meant that it was harder to prepare food. I was hungrier, but instead of seeking healthier options, I craved sugar, caffeine and junk food.

Less sleep = more hunger

The hormone ghrelin stimulates your appetite and promotes fat storage. Leptin suppresses your appetite and regulates the energy you expend. When both hormones are functioning correctly, they regulate normal feelings of hunger. When you do not get enough sleep, ghrelin levels increase and leptin levels decline, leaving you feeling hungry with an increased appetite.[85]

A lack of sleep also raises endocannabinoid levels. This makes the act of eating more enjoyable but also increases the desire for fatty food.[86] Studies have found that sleep-deprived people consume an extra 385 calories per day on average.[87] This is especially true when the time awake is spent being inactive.

We've seen the impact that a lack of good-quality sleep has. Now it is time to look at how to improve it.

The sleep cycle

On average, we spend one-third of our time on Planet Earth in the Land of Nod.[88] A poor night's sleep can leave us feeling worn out, emotional and fed up.[89] Sleep quality is as important as sleep quantity, and each stage of sleep has its benefits.

The four stages of sleep run in full cycles of roughly 90–110 minutes and are split into two phases: non-rapid eye movement (NREM) and rapid eye movement (REM). How long you spend in each depends on the time of night.

Let's look more closely at each stage of the sleep cycle.

Stage one (NREM)

This is the period between being awake and being asleep. Your brain activity starts to slow down, your body temperature drops, your muscles relax and you begin to lose awareness of your surroundings, but you'll still be easily awoken. If you've ever dozed off only to wake and claim to be 'resting your eyes', you were likely in stage one. Think of the person on the train who miraculously wakes up at their stop even though their head is bobbing. You may hallucinate while in this state – again, think of the person on the train who kicks their leg out and then wakes up a bit embarrassed.

This stage of sleep is one of the times when your mind is at its most creative. Some of the world's greatest minds have used this to their benefit. According to apocryphal legend, Albert Einstein would often sit in his favourite armchair and hold a pencil or spoon over a plate. When it fell, the noise would wake him instantly. He ensured he woke up before hitting stage two of sleep. In his wisdom, Einstein knew these micro naps, called hypnagogic naps, were critical for sharpening his mind long before science proved this theory.[90]

Stage two (NREM)

This stage is characterised by a slowing heart rate and a further decrease in body temperature. Your body reduces its activity as it prepares to go into the deepest part of sleep – stage three.

Stage three (NREM)

This is the deepest stage of sleep and waking up from this stage is rare.

This is when the body repairs tissues, boosts immune function and re-energises for the next day.

Stage four (REM)

As the name suggests, your eyes will move rapidly at this stage. This is when you dream most and your brain is most active. Your muscles are paralysed, stopping you from acting out your thoughts.

To ensure that we go through each stage, it's essential to have good sleep hygiene – to get everything in place to achieve optimal sleep.[91] Your pre-bed routine will have a big impact on your sleep quality, and this routine begins in the early evening.

The evening

Caffeine

Coffee shops in the city are full of eager punters waiting for their morning fix. The not-so-secret ingredient in coffee that gives you the edge is caffeine, a potent stimulant that works by attaching to adenosine receptors in your brain.

As soon as you wake up, adenosine starts dripping. As the day goes on, your brain's receptors are slowly filled, causing you to become sleepier until they're full – then you're ready for sleep. Caffeine works by binding to the adenosine receptors so that the adenosine can't work, halting the feeling of drowsiness.[92]

Imagine queuing to get into a bar, and when you get to the door, the bouncer tells you that the venue is full. When adenosine tries to bind to the receptors, they find out that they're full of caffeine and can't do so.

The problem is that although the club was full, it didn't stop the queue from forming at the door. As caffeine starts to leave, generally between 4–6 hours after entering, depending on how fast you metabolise it, adenosine starts to replace it. This is why when the caffeine wears off you may feel an intense wave of tiredness go through your body – all the adenosine rushes in at once.

Interestingly, adenosine is also believed to be involved in reducing neurotransmitters, including dopamine and adrenaline, so caffeine can also block this effect. This means that there will be more dopamine and your body is able to function at a higher level, which may help explain why caffeine is so addictive.[93]

You may notice over time that you need more caffeine to get the same effect. This is because your brain adapts to caffeine consumption by creating more receptors, so that there's more room for adenosine to attach – and it's why when you suddenly stop drinking caffeine, you may feel unpleasant withdrawal symptoms. With plenty of receptors and no competition, adenosine can work overtime, which may make you feel tired and depressed and even leave you with a banging headache. Fortunately, over time, the extra receptors will close.[94]

Caffeine is fine in moderation but can affect sleep when consumed later in the day. Drink your last cup at least 4–6 hours before you plan to sleep, to avoid disruption.[95]

Late-night exercise

Exercising intensely late in the evening can make it difficult for some people to fall asleep. However, a study published in *Sports Medicine* suggests that exercising in the evening is fine as long as you 'avoid vigorous activity for at least one hour before bedtime'. Exercising in the evening may even help you sleep better.[96]

If you're sensitive to the rush that comes with a challenging workout, you may want to exercise in the morning. If you prefer to exercise in the evenings, it's best to do so a few hours before bedtime and reduce the intensity of the workout.

Alcohol

It's easy to get into a routine of grabbing a nice bottle of red wine after a long, stressful day. A glass or two each evening can seemingly 'take the edge off', but it can also increase your stress levels the next day.

Alcohol helps you enter sleep faster but reduces your chances of entering REM sleep. It increases deep sleep during the first part of the night, but during the second part, this sleepy effect wears off and you'll be more likely to wake up or toss and turn, reducing your overall time spent asleep.

While this effect isn't significant when you consume low amounts of alcohol, moderate and high amounts cause an overall reduction in total REM percentage throughout the night.[97]

It can also lead you to wake up needing to pee. Your sleep will be broken, and it will be harder to enter deep sleep.

The last hour or two

In his insightful book *Why We sleep*, Mathew Walker suggests that keeping to a regular sleep cycle and going to bed and waking up at the same time each day, when possible, are the most important sleep habits to get a restful night.[98] This allows your body to maintain a regular sleep–wake cycle, which is regulated by a circadian rhythm. Your circadian rhythms are part of your internal clock, and they run on cycles that are roughly 24 hours. You may notice that your energy peaks and troughs throughout the day – this is because of your sleep cycle.[99]

Internal clocks that run fast or slow can result in disrupted or abnormal circadian rhythms. This can impact your hormone release, eating habits, digestion, body temperature and other bodily functions. Irregular rhythms have been linked to various chronic health conditions, such as sleep disorders, obesity, diabetes, depression, bipolar disorder and seasonal affective disorder.[100]

Regular sleep patterns can be challenging for those who have to travel to another time zone for work. Your biological clock will reset, but this often takes a few days, by which point you may already be on your way back to the previous time zone. When you do this regularly, it can play havoc on your sleep–wake cycle.

There are ways to reduce the effects of jet lag. Before your flight, gradually change your sleep routine – start going to bed and getting up an hour or two earlier or later than usual so that you begin to align with the time of your destination.

On the flight, try to avoid caffeine and alcohol and instead drink plenty of water. Only sleep if the flight matches the time for sleeping at your destination.

When you arrive, change your sleep pattern to match the new time zone as quickly as possible. To stay on local time, set your alarm to avoid oversleeping and go outside as soon as possible to get some natural light so that your body clock begins to adjust.

Exposing yourself to lots of bright light first thing will wake you up faster and improve your mood and alertness for the upcoming day. This is also why avoiding light before bed is so important.

Avoid bright light

When it's time for you to sleep, the hypothalamus, which controls your circadian rhythms, sends signals to your body to release melatonin, which makes you feel drowsy. However, any form of light can affect this.[101]

When light gets into your room (from a streetlight, for example), it can make your brain think that morning is coming. A pitch-black room will enable you stay in a deep sleep for longer.

Another form of light that can wreak havoc with sleep is the blue light emitted from smartphones, TVs and laptops. It can suppress the secretion of melatonin and reset your internal body clock so that you're more alert late at night.[102] This can be avoided by reducing your exposure to blue light at least 1 hour before bed. If you must work late using a computer, invest in blue light glasses.

EXERCISE

Try to avoid looking at your phone for the last hour before bedtime. Put the phone in another room until the morning. If you use it as an alarm clock, invest in a digital alarm clock to replace the need for the phone.

Take a hot bath and read a good book

Checking emails late at night will not only expose you to blue light but also keep your brain switched on. It's essential to allow yourself mental recovery during the day and also when you're trying to create an environment for a good night's sleep.

Although it can be hard to switch off, the work will still be there tomorrow, and you can only do so much each day. Your ability to get stuff done will only be reduced if you don't recover properly each night. Implementing a healthy nightly ritual will help you to fall asleep faster and to sleep deeper, so you recharge sufficiently for the next day.

A great way to set yourself up for a restful night is to enjoy a hot bath or shower before bedtime. Research suggests that it's best to have a bath between one and two hours before bed.[103] When your body temperature drops, your heart rate, breathing and digestion will slow, setting your body up nicely for optimal sleep. Even in the hotter months, a hot bath will help you sleep by raising your body temperature and then allowing it to cool after.

If this isn't possible – maybe you're arriving home late from the office and want to get straight into bed – running your wrists under hot water will give you similar benefits.

Add a good book to this routine and your brain will be able to completely switch off from the day's demands, and you'll enter a calm state much faster. Just 6 minutes of reading is shown to reduce stress by 68% and thus clearing the mind ready for sleep.[104]

Being too hot in bed can have the opposite effect and keep you up during the night.

Make your room a cave

Trying to sleep on a hot night can be frustrating and affect your sleep quality. Research shows that the optimal room temperature to get a great night's sleep is between 16°C and 18°C (60°F and 65°F). If your room is too warm, you're likely to have a restless night. A cold room may prevent you from nodding off easily.[105]

The final step

Sleep is essential for your mind and body. Improving your pre-bed routine will help you enjoy deeper and longer sleep. Although all these practices will afford you more recovery in your day-to-day life, there's something else you need to do: take an extended break. In the busy modern world, periods of complete downtime are vital. Try to give yourself an extended break every three months. This doesn't necessarily mean a full holiday – even three or four days will make all the difference. I've experienced the negative effects of going for too long without a break, despite having implemented all the previously mentioned practices.

Just as holidays are crucial to avoid burning out, rest weeks from working out are essential to allow your body to recover. This is known as de-loading, and the aim is to reduce the intensity and volume of your training. As a rough guide, you should de-load every twelve weeks.

Implementing recovery strategies into your life will enable you to perform at a high level. You'll be more energised, focused and driven during the day, you'll recover from workouts faster and you'll have fewer cravings for sugary treats, among many other benefits.

When you combine proper recovery with a smart exercise strategy and a well-balanced diet, you'll elevate your performance to a whole new level. Making all these elements work within your busy lifestyle is the final step.

Key points

- Your pre-bed ritual will have a big impact on how well you sleep. A structured routine will make you feel confident about your ability to have a restful night.

- Preparing for sleep starts well before bed. Limit your caffeine intake a minimum of 6 hours before you plan to sleep. Also limit your alcohol intake and avoid intense workouts right before bed.

- In the last hour or two before bed, begin unwinding by having a hot bath or shower and/or reading a good book. Make sure your room is dark and cool, and go to bed at roughly the same time each night.

PART THREE
MAKING IT HAPPEN

17
Your Transformational Journey

We've done a deep dive into the key areas that you need to focus on to achieve your peak mental and physical performance. However, there's an important factor that we've yet to discuss – how to get mentally prepared and ensure that the route you take on your transformational journey is efficient and effective.

This is where you take all the things you've learned in the previous chapters and make them work within your life.

Run your body as if it's a business

Incorporating exercise, healthier food choices and recovery into a busy schedule isn't easy; it requires you to plan ahead and create an environment that supports consistency. The strategy has many similarities to starting and running a business. Let's explore this idea.

Every successful business begins with the entrepreneur's vision. They may see a gap in the market and a problem that needs to be solved. There may be a cause behind the business. When you speak to them, they'll often be able to articulate where they want the business to go and why they're so passionate about it.

When starting a business, an entrepreneur understands that they're playing the long game. Although they'll need to turn over money quickly, the process of making the business a success is an ongoing one. Before launching, they'll create a strategy to begin the journey on the right foot. They'll evaluate the competition, do market research, and more, to ensure that the steps they take are logical. This won't guarantee them instant success, but they'll gain confidence that they're starting on the right track.

They'll add structure to look after the business's critical areas, including operations, marketing, sales and finances. Long-term targets in line with the bigger vision will be set. Objectives based on quarterly performance will also be set, allowing them to stay nimble and make changes to hit yearly targets.

Once they're confident that they have everything in place, they'll get the ball rolling by implementing the plan and testing it. After some time, they'll re-evaluate to see how they're doing. They'll make adjustments where necessary and test them as well.

Again, there's no guarantee of success, but by following a structured approach and getting into good habits, they increase their chances of it.

It would make no sense to leave things to chance. They cannot control the business environment, but they can control how they react to change by having systems and strategies in place.

Of course, not everybody takes this approach – and that's perhaps why 20% fail after their first year and 60% fail within their first three years.[106] Now consider the statistics around fitness goals. Up to 73% of people whose New Year's resolution is to get in shape give up before achieving their goals.[107]

There are many similarities between running a business and looking after your body.

Both are challenging and require a strategy and structure to increase the chances of success. You'll need to play the long game. That doesn't mean that you can't expect fast results, but it's essential to take the proper steps to make your changes sustainable. This means knowing where you are now, where you want to go and why you want to get there. You'll need to have a long-term goal, set quarterly objectives and use a system to ensure the changes you make work.

It begins by understanding why you're beginning your transformational journey.

The 5 whys

Have you ever considered your underlying reason behind wanting to get in shape? What's your deeper why?

I want to sit into a deep squat and do a pull-up when I'm eighty years old. That's my deeper reason.

Why is that important to me? Because I want to be fit, strong and mobile in later life.

Why is that important to me? Because I want to be able to play with my grandchildren when they're growing up.

I can keep peeling back the layers of why this is important to me, and the deeper I go, the more I identify with the outcome. This keeps me driven.

Others may want to lose weight because of something that happened in their childhood. Or maybe because they want to be a good role model for their children. Everyone has a different deeper why, but we all have one.

The deeper you dig into why you're beginning your transformational journey, the easier it is to focus when the initial motivation begins to fade. It may be the difference between persevering when times become tough or returning to old habits.

Developing a clear why is one of the most important steps you'll take on your transformational journey. It will allow you to remain focused on your outcome and driven to succeed even when times become challenging.

EXERCISE

Ask yourself this question: what is the underlying reason motivating me to change, and what am I aiming to achieve?

Consider your answer and why this is important to you. Then ask yourself why that is important to you. Repeat this process to uncover your deeper why.

> **FREE GIFT**
>
> Go to https://pathtopeakcondition.com/freegift to use our 5 Whys tool to dig deeper into your why.

Ideal outcome

Take a moment to consider what your ideal day would look like. Before you begin thinking about lying on golden sands in the Caribbean, I'll stop you and say that I mean your ideal 'normal' day. What routine would you follow from the moment you woke up until you went to bed so that you'd feel calm, focused, confident and happy? It doesn't matter how different it is from your routine now. Just imagine how you'd like to live, look and feel.

When we desire a lifestyle change – losing weight, getting fit or feeling stronger – we seek to move away from a current situation and towards a new experience.

You don't just want to lose weight; you want the feeling of losing weight. You don't just want the physical rewards of being fitter or stronger; you want the feeling of being fit and strong. You want to create a new identity. You want to be someone who is fitter and stronger, and to experience all the benefits that come with this.

Paint a picture of not only how you want to look and feel, but also the lifestyle you want to live. The more vivid the picture, the more real it becomes.

Ask yourself these questions:

- How do I want to look when I stand in front of the mirror naked? (Although body fat and weight are good markers to track progress, how we see ourselves when we look in the mirror is most important.)

- How do I want to look when I walk down the beach? How would looking this way make me feel?

- How many times a week do I want to work out? (Don't worry about the 'right' number. Focus on what would work for you and how it would make you feel.)

- How many times a week do I want to go out to eat and socialise? Does this match with the outcome I want? What would this look like in a perfectly balanced world?

- How many hours of good-quality sleep do I want to achieve? How would getting this sleep make me feel?

- What does my perfect pre-sleep ritual involve? How would I ensure I got a restful night?

- How many holidays do I want to take each year, and how many shorter breaks?

- What's a good balance between work and downtime on an average day? How would my day be structured to achieve it? How would this balance make me feel?

- What would my morning routine be like and why?

- How do I want to feel when I run, work out or play with young family members?

Some of the routines and outcomes you want may involve things that you used to do. People often say to me that they want to feel like themselves again. They've simply fallen into bad habits.

By defining the lifestyle you want to live, you can begin to build the habits needed to achieve that goal. Once you have a clear understanding of your why and the outcome you're aiming for, it's time to add definable landmarks to ensure you're on track to achieve it.

Landmark goals

In my experience as a coach, I've found that people who are getting married are among the most driven. They're focused on a specific date and will do whatever it takes to achieve their goal. The problems arise after they've reached their goal and the event has passed. All too often, they struggle to maintain momentum. The wedding is the end goal instead of a stepping-stone, so their journey ends there.

It's crucial to have a long-term landmark goal which ties in with your ideal outcome. Instead of looking at it as your end goal, though, see it as the first of many long-term targets you'll set on your transformational journey.

Just as a business will have yearly goals, so should you. Year on year, aim to adjust and improve your routine. You'll begin to achieve goals that would have been inconceivable at an earlier stage, and they'll become entirely expected.

For example, if one of your lifestyle goals is to run twice a week, then the landmark goal could be to run 10 miles at a speed of 10 minutes per mile by the end of the year. This won't happen on every run but will give you a target time and distance to aim for.

The clearer you become on each goal, the more exciting and realistic it will seem.

Although it's important to make each goal achievable, don't set the bar too low. Think of various successes you've achieved in life. They likely seemed impossible at first, but they became a reality because you kept taking deliberate actions towards them.

Before Roger Bannister ran a 4-minute mile in 1954, people thought it was impossible. At the time of writing, over 1,000 people have achieved this 'impossible' feat.[108]

Aim high – lofty ambitions lead to remarkable achievements.

Quarterly objectives

A year can seem a long way away, so aiming solely for a yearly goal can quickly lead to a loss of focus. This is why it's important to set quarterly objectives.

Many transformation programmes promise to get you the result you want, and then they finish. They do whatever it takes to help you achieve the desired outcome with little thought for what happens after, often leading to a return to old habits.

We all want to see fast results, but none of us wants to go back once we've hit our objective. The quarterly objective is simply a milestone on the way to a lifelong transformation. Keeping this in mind will ensure you don't take an unsustainable approach.

Break your one-year goal into four-quarters (about ninety days). Let's use the previous example of running 10 miles at a speed of 10 minutes per mile. For this scenario, let's imagine that when the goal was decided on, you were out of shape and struggled to run around the block. You'd likely find the idea of running 10 miles overwhelming. By breaking it down into quarterly objectives, the target will suddenly seem much more achievable.

The initial target could be to run nonstop for 2.5 miles by the end of the first quarter. Although still challenging, this is doable. You could then increase the distance by 2.5 miles every quarter. By the time the year mark came around, you'd be running 10 miles.

EXERCISE

What is your one-year goal?

Set a big goal and then split it into four stages. It will suddenly seem achievable.

FREE GIFT

Go to https://pathtopeakcondition.com/freegift for a free goal-setting document.

The last step is to begin ingraining the right habits to hit your quarterly goal – and there's an EASI way to do this.

EASI

Every lifestyle change begins with a spike in motivation, but this motivation lasts only for so long. Inevitably, it begins to fade, and this is when people tend to rely on willpower.

We all have willpower, but each of us has a limit. The more decisions you make, the faster willpower depletes. We use willpower throughout the day, for both straight-forward decisions, such as getting out of bed, and more testing ones, such as opting out of a debate with a fickle colleague. Each decision takes from the limited supply of willpower.

Think of it this way: when you use the same muscle during a workout session, that muscle will feel a greater level of fatigue. Every decision you make is essentially one more mental repetition.

This is why it's essential to remove as many decisions as possible regarding your health and fitness. The more you simplify the process, the greater your chance of adherence. You'll reduce your decision fatigue.

To achieve this, you need to know where to begin, what to adjust, how to structure your day and how to make sure that the strategy is effective. There's a four-step process you can follow, which I call EASI.

EASI is an acronym for evaluate, adjust, structure and implement. It's a simple and highly effective strategy for fine-tuning your routine so that it's efficient and allows you to create healthier lifestyle habits gradually.

You will have already begun painting a picture in your mind's eye of your perfect routine. This is the system that will allow you to make it a reality.

You'll use EASI to map out the best way to begin your journey and then reassess every two weeks after that. It's quick and easy and will transform your life.

First, let's look at evaluate.

Evaluate

As discussed, you're likely unaware of many of your daily habits. Exercise choices, food choices, what you do in the morning, before bed, during meetings, during periods in your week that are busier and periods that are quieter – many of these things will be automatic. This is what you're going to consider during your evaluation phase.

Look for trends that can be manipulated so that you can fit healthier alternatives into your day. Let's use the example of scheduling time to work out. Begin by looking at the general trends in your week, such as the days and times you have the most meetings, or when last-minute meetings are most commonly scheduled. Also, look at your energy levels during the day. If you feel tired in the evening but energised in the morning, it would be unwise to plan to exercise after work.

You'll begin to build a picture of your routine, and you may be surprised by what you find. It will give you a better understanding of where in your day you can schedule a time to exercise so you're unlikely to cancel.

This is the preparation phase. Get a bird's-eye view of your routine to find the best possible times to implement a new action, and highlight the areas where change will be easiest, so you see quick results.

The word *consistency* is bandied around in fitness. It's undoubtably necessary to see results and make them sustainable, but it's also one of the hardest things to achieve. If consistency were easy, everybody would be successful, but it is possible – and it requires a plan.

By evaluating your routine, you'll be able to see where you're being inconsistent. You'll find pockets of space in your day where you can implement a habit and remove obstacles that may be impeding your ability to live a happier, healthier and more productive life.

Adjust

Once you've been through the evaluation phase, it's time to think about how best to begin your journey. The aim is to make the smallest possible change to your routine and then continue to make small adjustments, so that you create momentum.

Again, let's use the example of creating an exercise habit. If you're not currently working out, then the process is simple – add one workout into your routine. Remember, make the process as easy as possible. You can always add more sessions when it has become routine, but you want to avoid going backwards.

Many people initially set the bar too high and then struggle to achieve their goal, which leaves them feeling as if they've failed, even though they're still doing better than they were.

For example, someone may get a hit of motivation to start working out. They decide to work out four times every week and hit this target for the first two weeks. Then the following week they do three sessions. The week after, two sessions. This creates the perception of losing momentum instead of gaining it.

Now say that same person decided to go to the gym once a week. They hit that target and decide that after working out on Monday, they feel good enough to go again on Thursday. Suddenly, they're overachieving and creating momentum. This simple change in mindset can have a massive difference in how they see the situation.

In his book, *Tiny Habits*, BJ Fogg talks about the smallest change possible to begin ingraining a new habit.[109] By starting with a smaller target, you ensure that you can remain consistent and progress over time. It's natural to want to do as much as possible in the hope of seeing faster results, but this journey is about making incremental improvements each day. An athlete doesn't begin their career by breaking world records. Most Hollywood actors don't have a blockbuster smash with their first acting role. An entrepreneur won't build a multimillion-pound company in weeks. All these people start small, learn as they go and become better over time. They build momentum.

We often look at what someone has achieved and forget about the journey they took to get there. Every outstanding achievement begins with a small action.

Remember, when making a lifestyle change, small and consistent beats significant and unsustainable. Aim for progress over quick wins.

Structure

With the information unearthed in the evaluation phase, you can structure new action into your routine. Without good structure, it will be difficult to remain consistent.

Imagine that you removed all the appointments and tasks from your diary for the upcoming week, but you still had to complete them. It's not likely you'd get everything done. Exercise, a balanced diet and recovery are no different – if you don't schedule them in advance, they likely won't happen. Yet, this is how many people approach their well-being. They fit a workout into their day when possible and grab food on the go.

It's crucial to plan ahead. In a perfect world, you'd aim to work out at roughly the same time and on the same days each week so that your workout would become a normal part of your routine. Once you find the best time, lock it into your diary and treat it as a high priority. Only cancel if you have no other choice. One missed session can easily turn into a few.

Of course, life changes. Sticking to the same times won't always be possible. Getting into a routine of checking your diary at the start of each week to see if anything could stop you from working out will allow you to make changes in advance.

Ask yourself these questions:

- Are my scheduled workout times appropriate this week?

- Is my workout location close and convenient?

- Do I have an exercise plan to follow?

- Is the duration of my workout appropriate for my schedule?

If there's a barrier stopping you from taking action, adjust the plan accordingly.

The second step is to make the process leading up to the workout as routine as possible. Remove the need to think, so that it becomes almost automatic.

Here are a few things to try:

- Prepare your clothes the night before and place them next to your front door, so they're ready to grab when you leave.

- Take the same route to your workout destination.

- If you go to a gym, use the same locker each time.

- Put on the same music as you start to exercise to create an association between that song and working out.

- When you finish, use the same shower cubicle and eat the same meal.

The more decisions you remove from your pre-workout routine, the quicker you'll create a lifestyle habit. The same is true for all of the habits we have discussed.

Lastly, it's time to implement and test.

Implement

After you implement your plan, test it for two weeks before making any changes. This timeframe will help you avoid being overreactive but will allow you to make changes if something clearly isn't working.

Every two weeks, look at how the biweekly targets worked within your routine:

- Did you hit all of them?

- Did you find them challenging?

- Are there better times that would work within your routine?

- Can you do more of what you're doing?

Over time, you'll better understand your routine and how to make adjustments. Keep adding more of the same actions until you find the sweet spot, but don't be tempted to move the process along too fast. Remember, it's better to continue making progress than to have to regress because you tried to move things along too fast.

At the same time, assess how you're progressing towards your exercise and aesthetic goals. Track your body statistics: your waist, hip, bicep and leg measurements, body weight and body fat percentage.

If measured on its own, weight can be a poor indicator of success unless you have a substantial amount to lose. Your weight can fluctuate by as much as 2.3–2.7 kg during the day. High stress levels, salt or a meal that's high in carbs can lead to water retention and impact your weight. Also, if you increase lean muscle while reducing overall body fat, your weight may not change at all. It's common to see people reduce their body fat or lose inches around their waist but stay about the same weight. Measuring weight alone can be demotivating and leave you feeling as if you're not making progress when you are.

Also, take a photo every few weeks. There's no better marker of success. Many people dislike taking a photo of themselves in their underwear, but it feels fantastic to look at a before picture and be able to see the change in your body.

Keep a log of your workouts and step count so that you can view your progress and adapt it depending on the results you see every two weeks. Remember to regularly assess your food diary.

Every time you achieve your biweekly target, celebrate it. Start small and build momentum. Harness that feeling of success to help create a winning mentality. Each time you achieve a target, you'll get a hit of dopamine, which is released when we do things that give us pleasure. When you add the endorphin high that comes from exercising into the mix, you'll suddenly be buzzing with an exercise-induced cocktail of feel-good chemicals. The best part is that this cocktail is free, legal and healthy.

Use EASI when implementing any of the nine habits into your routine. First, evaluate your routine to find the best time to add the habit. Make a small adjustment to avoid overwhelm and add structure to your day based on what you learned in the evaluation stage, before implementing and testing. Every two weeks, go through the same process: re-evaluate, make small adjustments, restructure if necessary, then implement and test.

If you continue to follow this process you will find the most time-efficient and effective strategy to transform how you look, feel and perform.

Key points

- Making a lifestyle change is tough. It requires planning, a strategy and structure. There are many similarities between looking after your body and running a successful business.

- Before you start your transformational journey, it's crucial to identify your deeper reason for taking the journey and the ideal outcome that you're aiming for. This will keep you driven when motivation is low.

- It's important to set long-, medium- and short-term targets to ensure you remain focused and on the right track. Plan where you want to be in one year and then break this down into quarterly objectives. Lastly, set yourself biweekly action-based targets and continually evaluate and adjust and restructure if necessary, before implementing and testing the changes. This way, you'll always be refining your approach so that it's time-efficient and effective.

Conclusion

Expected slips

Progress is important, but making a lifestyle change takes time and won't come without its setbacks. We are all human, and we all make mistakes. The way that we react to them is an essential part of maintaining a healthy lifestyle.

You know how it can happen. You make a promise to yourself to avoid eating a particular food, or to not drink alcohol, but your resolve breaks down and you indulge. Afterwards, you feel as if you've let yourself and others down, and you start to beat yourself up.

Instead of doing this, simply set the lapse aside, forget about it and try to go longer until you do it again. You're not a machine, so don't try to act like one. Accept your flaws, try to keep improving and move on.

Reward good behaviour and learn from the lapses. Focus on the good things you're achieving, and you'll end up doing more of them. Over time, you'll create lifelong habits.

Someone who plays golf vs a golfer

I play golf, but I'm not a golfer. The difference is important. I enjoy a round of golf every so often and pop over to the driving range if I have some free time, but if it's raining or a more attractive offer comes up, I might change my plans. A golfer, however, will prioritise golf over pretty much anything: if it's raining and cold, they still play.

In a golfer's mind, the sport is part of their very being. It's part of who they are. A golfer gets so much fulfilment and enjoyment from seeing progression in their game that they want to keep practising. They go to bed thinking about swinging that club, putting the ball and the feeling they'll get from beating an opponent who was once so much better than they were. If they can't play for a while, they'll continue thinking about golf and, when the time comes, they'll get straight back into 'the swing of it'.

The key to becoming a good golfer is to keep at it long enough that the upside outweighs the downside. When you start to play golf, it's tremendously frustrating; just hitting the ball is difficult, let alone aiming at a target. Many people quickly lose interest, but for those who continue past that initial phase and dedicate time to becoming a better player, the rewards are great.

If you speak to a golfer, they'll do their best to persuade you to take it up. They'll explain that it's frustrating at the start and tell you how they got through that first challenging period because they'll want you to enjoy the benefits that they do.

When we find something that's good, we want to tell others about it. We want them to experience the same buzz. Just as a golfer will try to persuade you to take up golf, someone who looks after their health and fitness will try to convince you to work out and eat well. They understand that the first phase is challenging – any new experience will test you – but they also know that the rewards far outweigh the effort.

The key is to hang in there long enough to get better, so the changes become part of your routine. Getting in shape takes time and repeated efforts. You don't need to be good initially. You should expect to find it challenging and frustrating, and you'll have to make a concerted effort, but it gets easier and becomes enjoyable.

Feeling better, well, feels good. You'll want more. Instead of forcing yourself to work out, eat nutritious food, go for that walk or get an early night, you'll want to. It will feel wrong not to. It will become part of your very being.

And you'll keep getting better. You'll shift from trying to get into shape to being in great shape. You won't attempt to achieve your ideal weight; you'll live with your perfect weight. You won't need to drag yourself out of bed; you'll bounce out ready for the day.

You'll look better, feel better and perform better. You'll be a better parent, partner and colleague. You'll be happier, healthier and more vibrant. What's perhaps most unbelievable is that you'll forget what things were like before you started. You'll wonder why you didn't start earlier. You'll become that person who tells others about the benefits and tries to persuade them to start.

No matter where you are on your fitness journey, the process never changes. The priority is to find the routine that works best within your life now. Keep adapting it so that making healthier food choices is easy; so that you work out at the most convenient time for you; so that you have time to go for a long, relaxing walk; so that you have a structured and empowering morning routine; so that your nightly ritual is conducive to a great night's sleep.

Life is constantly changing. Tomorrow will be different from today, and the day after that will be a whole new experience. All you can do is make sure that your routines, rituals and habits are set up to allow you to thrive in any situation.

Exercise, nutrition and recovery aren't just wellness strategies – they are a fundamental part of being happy. Life is better and more fulfilling when we're physically active, eat a well-rounded diet, have mental downtime and get a good night's sleep.

The fact that you've taken the time to read this book shows that you're already on the right track and ready to take action. Implementation is the key.

The order is important

There's a lot of information in this book, and you might not know where to start. If so, I suggest focusing on exercise and nutrition to begin with. This will get you the fastest return on your investment of time and effort.

Your body composition, fitness level and strength will improve. Also, as a result, your sleep quality will be better, and you'll get more mental downtime.

Once you've seen improvements in your diet and exercise routine for an extended period, begin focusing on recovery strategies. At this point, you'll feel so much better that it will be easier to make more changes.

Act today

Making what you've learned in this book work within your life might seem like a big task. Maybe you think that you don't have time, or that you're too busy to start at the moment and will begin next week.

Most people just keep waiting for the right moment but never act. They don't have enough energy, work is too busy or they believe that they don't have enough time to remain consistent. Don't wait for the green light to shine – this might never happen. Jump the light and start driving towards your goals now.

You have everything you need to transform how you look, feel and perform. Take control of the outcome and work towards the best version of you.

No matter your starting point, just make a small commitment. Perform one short workout, schedule time for a daily walk or start tracking what you eat. Now. Not tomorrow, or the day after.

One step turns into two, and your efforts will quickly compound. Focus on consistency, not quick wins. You're on a journey – there's no end point, just landmarks along the way.

As you integrate more healthy habits into your life, other aspects of this book will become relevant. It's best read a number of times. Use it as a reference, so that you're always progressing.

Good mental and physical well-being are true gifts that we must cherish. Look after them, protect them and enjoy them.

Small steps lead to big strides. Take your first today.

Extra reading

Many books have changed the way I see the world of health and well-being, and they prompted me to deep dive into extra research. You can find my recommended reading list at www.pathtopeakcondition.com /extrareading.

Resources

There are several resources that will help you reach your peak condition.

Reach Your Peak Quiz

This set of questions is based on the three core lifestyle habits described in this book. You'll be sent a customised report showing you where you're already strong and what areas you need to work on the most.

You can take fill out the scorecard at https://reachyourpeakquiz.com

Turning Point Sessions

Each week, I host Turning Point Sessions for a small number of people to help them implement the principles in this book.

Go to https://calendly.com/pathtopeakcondition /turningpointsession to book your space.

Path to Peak Condition Mastermind Facebook Group

Join our group and connect with other professionals and entrepreneurs. Get exclusive advice on exercise, nutrition and recovery from our expert coaches, and enjoy accountability and support from peers on a similar journey. Go to www.facebook.com/groups /pathtopeakcondition to join.

Path to Peak Condition Programme

The Path to Peak Condition Programme is a 52-week programme designed to help busy professionals and entrepreneurs make healthier lifestyle choices. Through the programme, you'll implement the nine core habits covered in this book, connect with a peer group on a similar journey, and work with our world-class coaches and dietitians.

For more information on the Path to Peak Condition Programme, go to https://pathtopeakcondition.com.

Notes

1. Society for Personality and Social Psychology, 'How we form habits, change existing ones', *ScienceDaily* (8 August 2014), www.sciencedaily.com/releases/2014/08/140808111931.htm
2. D Kahneman, *Thinking, Fast and Slow* (Penguin, 2011)
3. C Duhigg, *The Power of Habit* (Random House, 2012)
4. 'Calories burned in 30 minutes for people of three different weights', Harvard Health Publishing (8 March 2021), www.health.harvard.edu/diet-and-weight-loss/calories-burned-in-30-minutes-for-people-of-three-different-weights
5. P McCall, '7 things to know about excess post-exercise oxygen consumption (EPOC)' (The American Council on Exercise, 28 August 2014), www.acefitness.org/education-and-resources/professional/expert-articles/5008/7-things-to-know-about-excess-post-exercise-oxygen-consumption-epoc
6. J LaForgia, RT Withers and CJ Gore, 'Effects of exercise intensity and duration on the excess post-exercise oxygen consumption', *Journal of Sports Science*, 24/12 (2016), https://pubmed.ncbi.nlm.nih.gov/17101527
7. 'Brits lose count of their calories: Over a third of Brits don't know how many calories they consume on a typical day' (Mintel Press Office, 9 March 2016), www.mintel.com/press-centre/food-and-drink/brits-lose-count-of-their-calories-over-a-third-of-brits-dont-know-how-many-calories-they-consume-on-a-typical-day
8. C Baker, 'Obesity statistics' (House of Commons Library, 11 January 2021), https://commonslibrary.parliament.uk/research-briefings/sn03336
9. 'Scale of the obesity problem', *Health Matters: Obesity and the food environment* (Public Health England, 31 March 2017),

www.gov.uk/government/publications/health-matters-obesity
-and-the-food-environment/health-matters-obesity-and-the-food
-environment--2

10. T Mann, 'Why do dieters regain weight? Calorie deprivation
alters body and mind, overwhelming willpower' (American
Psychological Association, 2018), www.apa.org/science/about/psa
/2018/05/calorie-deprivation

11. A Keys et al, *The Biology of Human Starvation*, vols 1–2 (University
of Minnesota Press, 1950)

12. GD Foster et al, 'What is a reasonable weight loss? Patients'
expectations and evaluations of obesity treatment outcomes',
Journal of Consulting and Clinical Psychology, 65/1 (1997), https://
pubmed.ncbi.nlm.nih.gov/9103737

13. H Selye, *The Stress of Life* (McGraw-Hill, 1956)

14. J Berry, 'Endorphins: Effects and how to increase levels', *Medical
News Today* (6 February 2018), www.medicalnewstoday.com
/articles/320839

15. A Dietrich and WF McDaniel, 'Endocannabinoids and exercise',
British Journal of Sports Medicine, 38/5 (2004), https://bjsm.bmj.com
/content/38/5/536

16. Les Mills, 'Media release: Study sparks call for guidelines around
high-intensity interval training', *Fit Planet* (5 June 2018), www
.lesmills.com/uk/fit-planet/media/hiit-research

17. BA Roy, 'Overreaching/overtraining', *ACSM's Health and Fitness
Journal*, 19/2 (April 2015), https://journals.lww.com/acsm
-healthfitness/fulltext/2015/03000/overreaching_overtraining
__more_is_not_always.4.aspx

18. L Smith et al, 'Occupational physical activity habits of UK office
workers: Cross-sectional data from the active buildings study',
International Journal of Environmental Research and Public Health,
15/6 (2018), www.ncbi.nlm.nih.gov/pmc/articles/PMC6025535

19. SH Kang et al, 'Effect of sedentary time on the risk of orthopaedic
problems in people aged 50 years and older', *The Journal of
Nutrition, Health and Aging*, 24 (2020), https://link.springer.com
/article/10.1007/s12603-020-1391-7

20. 'Back pain experienced more frequently in the UK' (British
Chiropractic Association, 2020), https://chiropractic-uk.co.uk
/back-pain-experienced-frequently-uk

21. F Maij, AM Wing and WP Medendorp, 'Afferent motor feedback
determines the perceived location of tactile stimuli in the external
space presented to the moving arm', *Journal of Neurophysiology*,
118/1 (2017), www.ncbi.nlm.nih.gov/pmc/articles/PMC5494371

22. A Spina, 'Functional range conditioning' (FRS, no date), https://
functionalanatomyseminars.com/frs-system/functional-range
-conditioning

23. K Keller and M Engelhardt, 'Strength and muscle mass loss with aging process: Age and strength loss', *Muscles, Ligaments and Tendons Journal*, 3/4 (2013), www.ncbi.nlm.nih.gov/pmc/articles/PMC3940510

24. RR Kalyani, M Corriere and L Ferrucci, 'Age-related and disease-related muscle loss: The effect of diabetes, obesity and other diseases', *The Lancet Diabetes and Endocrinology*, 2/10 (2014), www.ncbi.nlm.nih.gov/pmc/articles/PMC4156923

25. 'Osteoporosis' (NHS, last reviewed 2019), www.nhs.uk/conditions/osteoporosis

26. T Sözen, L Özışık and N Başaran, 'An overview and management of osteoporosis', *European Journal of Rheumatology*, 4/1 (2017), pp46–56, https://doi.org/10.5152/eurjrheum.2016.048

27. 'Strength training: Get stronger, leaner, healthier' (Mayo Clinic, 2021), www.mayoclinic.org/healthy-lifestyle/fitness/in-depth/strength-training/art-20046670

28. BJ Schoenfeld, 'The mechanisms of muscle hypertrophy and their application to resistance training', *Journal of Strength and Conditioning Research*, 24/10 (2010), pp2857–2872, https://doi.org/10.1519/JSC.0b013e3181e840f3

29. BJ Schoenfeld, 'Potential mechanisms for a role of metabolic stress in hypertrophic adaptations to resistance training', *Sports Medicine*, 43/3 (2013), pp179–194, https://doi.org/10.1007/s40279-013-0017-1

30. NA Burd et al, 'Muscle time under tension during resistance exercise stimulates differential muscle protein sub-fractional synthetic responses in men', *The Journal of Physiology*, 590/2 (2012) pp351–362, https://doi.org/10.1113/jphysiol.2011.221200

31. M Krzysztofik et al, 'Maximizing muscle hypertrophy: A systematic review of advanced resistance training techniques and methods', *International Journal of Environmental Research and Public Health*, 16/24 (2019), https://doi.org/10.3390/ijerph16244897

32. F Damas, CA Libardi and C Ugrinowitsch, 'The development of skeletal muscle hypertrophy through resistance training: The role of muscle damage and muscle protein synthesis', *European Journal of Applied Physiology*, 118/3 (2018), https://doi.org/10.1007/s00421-017-3792-9

33. GA Borg, 'Perceived exertion as an indicator of somatic stress', *Scandinavian Journal of Rehabilitation Medicine*, 2/2 (1970), pp92–98

34. M Tuchscherer, *The Reactive Training Manual: Developing your own custom training program for powerlifting: reactive training systems* (self-published, 2008)

35. M Ormsbee et al, 'Efficacy of the repetitions in reserve-based rating of perceived exertion for the bench press in experienced and novice benchers', *Journal of Strength and Conditioning Research*, 33/2 (2019), https://pubmed.ncbi.nlm.nih.gov/28301439

36. JA Sampson and H Groeller, 'Failure is not necessary for strength gain', *Scandinavian Journal of Medicine and Science in Sports*, 26 (2016), https://doi.org/10.1111/sms.12445

37. J Steele at al, 'Ability to predict repetitions to momentary failure is not perfectly accurate, though improves with resistance training experience,' *PeerJ*, 5/e4105 (2017), www.ncbi.nlm.nih.gov/pmc/articles/PMC5712461

38. RR Wolfe, 'Fat metabolism in exercise', *Advances in Experimental Medicine and Biology*, 441 (1998), https://pubmed.ncbi.nlm.nih.gov/9781322

39. CE Kline, 'The bidirectional relationship between exercise and sleep: Implications for exercise adherence and sleep improvement', *American Journal of Lifestyle Medicine*, 8/6 (2015), www.ncbi.nlm.nih.gov/pmc/articles/PMC4341978

40. DL Tomlin and HA Wenger, 'The relationship between aerobic fitness and recovery from high intensity intermittent exercise', *Sports Medicine*, 31/1 (2001), https://pubmed.ncbi.nlm.nih.gov/11219498

41. Ibid

42. LH Willis et al, 'Effects of aerobic and/or resistance training on body mass and fat mass in overweight or obese adults', *Journal of Applied Physiology*, 113/12 (2012), https://doi.org/10.1152/japplphysiol.01370.2011

43. S Kai et al, 'Effectiveness of moderate-intensity interval training as an index of autonomic nervous activity', *Rehabilitation Research and Practice* (November 2016), www.ncbi.nlm.nih.gov/pmc/articles/PMC5121464; RB Wichi et al, 'A brief review of chronic exercise intervention to prevent autonomic nervous system changes during the aging process', *Clinics*, 64/3 (2009), www.ncbi.nlm.nih.gov/pmc/articles/PMC2666449

44. TL Fazzino, K Rohde and DK Sullivan, 'Hyper-palatable foods: Development of a quantitative definition and application to the US Food System Database', *Obesity (Silver Spring)*, 27/11 (2019), https://pubmed.ncbi.nlm.nih.gov/31689013

45. LR Young and M Nestle, (Feb 2003) 'Expanding portion sizes in the US marketplace: Implications for nutrition counselling', *Journal of the American Dietetic Association*, 103/2 (2003), https://pubmed.ncbi.nlm.nih.gov/12589331

46. PM Zuraikat et al, 'Increasing the size of portion options affects intake but not portion selection at a meal', *Appetite*, 98 (2016), www.ncbi.nlm.nih.gov/pmc/articles/PMC4728005

47. Kaiser Permanente, 'Keeping a food diary doubles diet weight loss, study suggests', *ScienceDaily* (8 July 2008), www.sciencedaily.com/releases/2008/07/080708080738.htm

48. H Harper and M Hallsworth, *Counting Calories: How under-reporting can explain the apparent fall in calorie intake* (Behavioural

Insights Team, 2016), www.bi.team/publications/counting
-calories-how-under-reporting-can-explain-the-apparent-fall-in
-calorie-intake.wpengine.netdna-cdn.com/wp-content/uploads
/2016/08/16-07-12-Counting-Calories-Final.pdf

49. CM Champagne et al, 'Energy intake and energy expenditure: A
controlled study comparing dietitians and non-dietitians', *Journal
of the American Dietetic Association*, 102/10 (2002), https://pubmed
.ncbi.nlm.nih.gov/12396160

50. S Lang, '"Mindless autopilot" drives people to dramatically
underestimate how many daily food decisions they make, Cornell
study finds', *Cornell Chronicle* (22 December 2006), https://news
.cornell.edu/stories/2006/12/mindless-autopilot-drives-people
-underestimate-food-decisions

51. See eg B Strasser, A Spreitzer and P Haber, (2007) 'Fat loss
depends on energy deficit only, independently of the method
for weight loss', *Annals of Nutrition and Metabolism*, 51/5 (2007),
pp428–432, https://doi.org/10.1159/000111162; I Romieu et al,
'Energy balance and obesity: What are the main drivers?' *Cancer
Causes Control*, 28 (2017), pp247–258, https://doi.org/10.1007/s10552
-017-0869-z; JO Hill et al, 'The importance of energy balance,'
European Endocrinology, 9/2 (2013), pp111-115, www.ncbi.nlm.nih
.gov/pmc/articles/PMC6003580

52. *Guidance for Industry: Guide for developing and using data bases
for nutrition labeling* (FDA, 1998), www.fda.gov/regulatory
-information/search-fda-guidance-documents/guidance-industry
-guide-developing-and-using-data-bases-nutrition-labeling

53. JA Whitworth, GJ Mangos and JJ Kelly, 'Cushing, cortisol, and
cardiovascular disease', *Hypertension*, 36/5 (1979), https://doi.org
/10.1161/01.hyp.36.5.912

54. R Schnepper et al, 'A combined mindfulness prolonged
chewing intervention reduces body weight, food craving, and
emotional eating, *Journal of Consulting and Clinical Psychology*,
87/1 (2019), www.researchgate.net/publication/330043007
_A_Combined_Mindfulness'Prolonged_Chewing_Intervention
_Reduces_Body_Weight_Food_Craving_and_Emotional_Eating

55. EM Blass, 'On the road to obesity: Television viewing increases
intake of high-density foods', *Physiology and Behavior*, 88/4–5,
pp597–604, https://pubmed.ncbi.nlm.nih.gov/16822530

56. DL Ballor et al, 'Resistance weight training during caloric
restriction enhances lean body weight maintenance', *The American
Journal of Clinical Nutrition*, 47/1 (1988), https://pubmed.ncbi.nlm
.nih.gov/3337037

57. TB Chaston, JB Dixon and PE O'Brien, 'Changes in fat-free mass
during significant weight loss: a systematic review', *International
Journal of Obesity*, 31/5 (2007), https://pubmed.ncbi.nlm.nih.gov
/17075583

58. RW Morton et al, 'A systematic review, meta-analysis and meta-regression of the effect of protein supplementation on resistance training-induced gains in muscle mass and strength in healthy adults', *British Journal of Sports Medicine*, 52/6 (2018), pp376–384, https://pubmed.ncbi.nlm.nih.gov/28698222

59. KR Westerterp, 'Diet induced thermogenesis', *Nutrition and Metabolism*, 1/5 (2004), www.ncbi.nlm.nih.gov/pmc/articles /PMC524030

60. DT Villareal et al, 'Effect of weight loss on the rate of muscle protein synthesis during fasted and fed conditions in obese older adults', *Obesity*, 20/9 (2012), pp1780–6, www.ncbi.nlm.nih.gov /pmc/articles/PMC3291735

61. The National Weight Control Registry (NWCR): www.nwcr.ws

62. DM Ostendorf et al, 'Physical activity energy expenditure and total daily energy expenditure in successful weight loss maintainers', *Obesity*, 27/3 (2019), pp496–504, https://pubmed.ncbi .nlm.nih.gov/30801984

63. ML Brandt, 'Pedometers help people count steps to get healthy', *Stanford News* (28 November 2007), https://news.stanford.edu /news/2007/november28/med-pedometer-112807.html

64. C Tudor-Locke and DR Bassett, 'How many steps/day are enough? Preliminary pedometer indices for public health', *Sports Medicine*, 34/1 (2004), https://pubmed.ncbi.nlm.nih.gov/14715035

65. KD Hall et al, 'Ultra-processed diets cause excess calorie intake and weight gain: An inpatient randomized controlled trial of ad libitum food intake', *Cell Metabolism*, 30/1 (2019), https://pubmed .ncbi.nlm.nih.gov/31105044

66. WC Willett, 'The Mediterranean diet: Science and practice,' *Public Health Nutrition*, 9/1A (2006), https://doi.org/10.1079/PHN2005931

67. A Trichopoulou et al, 'Adherence to a Mediterranean diet and survival in a Greek population', *The New England Journal of Medicine*, 26/348 (2003), www.nejm.org/doi/pdf/10.1056 /nejmoa025039

68. CD Gardner et al, 'Effect of low-fat vs low-carbohydrate diet on 12-month weight loss in overweight adults and the association with genotype pattern or insulin secretion: The DIETFITS randomized clinical trial', *JAMA*, 319/7 (2018), https:// jamanetwork.com/journals/jama/fullarticle/2673150

69. National Research Council (US) Committee on Diet and Health, *Diet and Health: Implications for Reducing Chronic Disease Risk* (National Academies Press, 1989), https://doi.org/10.17226/19023

70. NA Shaheen et al, 'Public knowledge of dehydration and fluid intake practices: variation by participants' characteristics', *BMC Public Health*, 18 (2018), www.ncbi.nlm.nih.gov/pmc/articles /PMC6282244; Georgia Institute of Technology, 'As we get parched, cognition can sputter, dehydration study says', *Newswise*

(17 July 2018), www.newswise.com/articles/as-we-get-parched
%2C-cognition-can-sputter%2C-dehydration-study-says

71. University of Birmingham, 'Glass of water before each meal could help in weight reduction', *Science Daily* (26 August 2015), www.sciencedaily.com/releases/2015/08/150826101645.htm

72. H Mills, N Reiss and M Dombeck, 'Mental and emotional impact of stress', Helen Farabee Centers (no date), www.helenfarabee.org/poc/view_doc.php?type=doc&id=15649&cn=117

73. Ibid

74. J MacKay, 'Screen time stats 2019: Here's how much you use your phone during the workday', *RescueTime: blog* (21 March 2019), https://blog.rescuetime.com/screen-time-stats-2018

75. P Burgess et al, 'Stress management: Breathing exercises for relaxation (University of Michigan Health, 31 August 2020), www.uofmhealth.org/health-library/uz2255

76. Trinity College Dublin, 'The Yogi masters were right – meditation and breathing exercises can sharpen your mind: New research explains link between breath-focused meditation and attention to brain health', *ScienceDaily* (10 May 2018), www.sciencedaily.com/releases/2018/05/180510101254.htm

77. 'The process of breathing' (Lumen Learning, no date), https://courses.lumenlearning.com/suny-ap2/chapter/the-process-of-breathing-no-content

78. J Gifford, 'The secret of the 10% most productive people? Breaking!', *DeskTime* (14 May 2018), https://desktime.com/blog/17-52-ratio-most-productive-people

79. M Oppezzo and DL Schwartz, 'Give your ideas some legs: The positive effect of walking on creative thinking', *Journal of Experimental Psychology*, 40/4 (2014), www.apa.org/pubs/journals/releases/xlm-a0036577.pdf

80. 'Vitamin D' (Heart UK, no date), www.heartuk.org.uk/low-cholesterol-foods/vitamin-d

81. I Anjum et al, 'The role of vitamin D in brain health: A mini literature review', *Cureus*, 10/7 (2018), www.ncbi.nlm.nih.gov/pmc/articles/PMC6132681

82. N Rose, *Churchill: The Unruly Giant* (Simon & Schuster, 1995)

83. B Rasch and J Born, 'About sleep's role in memory', *Physiological Reviews*, 93/2 (2013), www.ncbi.nlm.nih.gov/pmc/articles/PMC3768102

84. J Underwood, *Sleep and Recovery* (Life of an Athlete, 2018), www.wm.edu/offices/sportsmedicine/_documents/sleep-manual

85. S Taheri et al, 'Short Sleep Duration Is Associated with Reduced Leptin, Elevated Ghrelin, and Increased Body Mass Index', *PLoS Medicine*, 1/3 (2004), www.ncbi.nlm.nih.gov/pmc/articles/PMC535701

86. EC Hanlon et al, 'Sleep restriction enhances the daily rhythm of circulating levels of endocannabinoid 2-arachidonoylglycerol', *Sleep*, 39/3 (2016), www.ncbi.nlm.nih.gov/pmc/articles /PMC4763355

87. King's College London, 'Sleep deprivation may cause people to eat more calories', *ScienceDaily* (2 November 2016), www.sciencedaily .com/releases/2016/11/161102130724.htm

88. MJ Aminoff, F Boller and DF Swaab, 'We spend about one-third of our life either sleeping or attempting to do so', *Handbook of Clinical Neurology*, 98/7 (2011), https://pubmed.ncbi.nlm.nih.gov/21056174

89. HK Al Khatib et al, 'The effects of partial sleep deprivation on energy balance: A systematic review and meta-analysis', *European Journal of Clinical Nutrition*, 71/5 (2017), https://pubmed.ncbi.nlm .nih.gov/27804960

90. 'Famous nappers: Albert Einstein, Salvador Dali, Bill Clinton go to bed to get ahead', *Herald Sun* (17 December 2014), www.heraldsun.com.au/news/victoria/famous-nappers-albert -einstein-salvador-dali-bill-clinton-go-to-bed-to-get-ahead/news -story/8e764c1d50a13d122641bcbd4086624d

91. 'Sleep basics' (Cleveland Clinic, reviewed 7 December 2020), https://my.clevelandclinic.org/health/articles/12148-sleep-basics

92. M Lazarus et al, 'Arousal effect of caffeine depends on adenosine A2A receptors in the shell of the nucleus accumbens', *Journal of Neuroscience*, 31/27 (2011), www.ncbi.nlm.nih.gov/pmc/articles /PMC3153505

93. ND Valkow et al, 'Caffeine increases striatal dopamine D2/D3 receptor availability in the human brain', *Translational Psychiatry*, 5/4 (2015), www.ncbi.nlm.nih.gov/pmc/articles/PMC4462609/ #__sec1title

94. JP Boulenger et al, 'Chronic caffeine consumption increases the number of brain adenosine receptors', *Life Sciences*, 32/10 (1983), https://pubmed.ncbi.nlm.nih.gov/6298543

95. 'Spilling the beans: How much caffeine is too much?' (US Food and Drug Administration, 12 December 2018), www.fda.gov /consumers/consumer-updates/spilling-beans-how-much -caffeine-too-much

96. J Stutz, R Eiholzer and CM Spengler, 'Effects of evening exercise on sleep in healthy participants: A systematic review and meta-analysis', *Sports Medicine*, 49 (2019), https://link.springer.com /article/10.1007/s40279-018-1015-0

97. MM Thakkar, R Sharma and P Sahota, 'Alcohol disrupts sleep homeostasis', *Alcohol*, 49/4 (2015), https://pubmed.ncbi.nlm.nih .gov/25499829

98. M Walker, *Why We Sleep: the new science of sleep and dreams* (Penguin, 2018)

99. J-H Kang and S-C Chen, 'Effects of an irregular bedtime schedule on sleep quality, daytime sleepiness, and fatigue among university students in Taiwan', *BMC Public Health*, 9 (2009), www.ncbi.nlm.nih.gov/pmc/articles/PMC2718885

100. S Reddy, V Reddy and S Sharma, 'Physiology, circadian rhythm', *StatPearls* (January 2001), www.ncbi.nlm.nih.gov/books/NBK519507

101. JJ Gooley et al, 'Exposure to room light before bedtime suppresses melatonin onset and shortens melatonin duration in humans', *The Journal of Clinical Endocrinology and Metabolism*, 96/3 (2011), www.ncbi.nlm.nih.gov/pmc/articles/PMC3047226

102. 'Blue light has a dark side' (Harvard Health Publishing, 7 July 2020), www.health.harvard.edu/staying-healthy/blue-light-has-a-dark-side

103. S Haghayegh et al, 'Before-bedtime passive body heating by warm shower or bath to improve sleep: A systematic review and meta-analysis', *Sleep Medicine Reviews*, 46 (2019), www.sciencedirect.com/science/article/abs/pii/S1087079218301552

104. D Lewis, 'Reading can help reduce stress', *The Telegraph* (30 March 2009), www.telegraph.co.uk/news/health/news/5070874/Reading-can-help-reduce-stress.html

105. N Silver, 'What is the best temperature for sleep?', *Healthline* (13 December 2019), www.healthline.com/health/sleep/best-temperature-to-sleep

106. '60% of new businesses fail in the first 3 years: Here's why', *Durham City Incubator* (7 November 2019), https://dcincubator.co.uk/blog/60-of-new-businesses-fail-in-the-first-3-years-heres-why

107. 'New study finds 73% of people who set fitness goals as new year's resolutions give them up', Bodybuilding.com (9 January 2019), www.bodybuilding.com/fun/2013-100k-transformation-contest-press-release.html

108. B Taylor, 'What breaking the 4-minute mile taught us about the limits of conventional thinking', *Harvard Business Review* (9 March 2018), https://hbr.org/2018/03/what-breaking-the-4-minute-mile-taught-us-about-the-limits-of-conventional-thinking

109. BJ Fogg, *Tiny Habits: The small changes that change everything* (Houghton Mifflin Harcourt, 2019)

Acknowledgements

Thanks to Neil and Mary McIntosh, Florian Weber, Michele Reedy, Ian Thomas, Sally Clark, Andy Crispin, Pedro Dias Ferreira, Steve Frost, James Corrales and Damien O'Dwyer for taking the time to read the manuscript and give your valued feedback at different stages of writing.

Thanks to every client I've coached for giving me a chance to work with you and test the ideas and systems within this book.

Lastly, thanks to my mother, father and stepfather for helping me grow as a person.

The Author

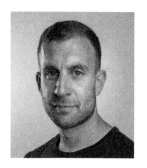

Alex Pedley is a personal trainer, entrepreneur and speaker. Over the last two decades, he has clocked up tens of thousands of coaching hours working with professionals from all corners of the business world, including high-profile CEOs, bankers and lawyers.

Alex is the founder of the Alex Pedley Academy, which offers transformation accelerators for busy professionals. The academy shows high performers how to implement nine core habits into their lives, so that they look better, feel better and perform better.

Alex regular speaks to international corporations on the topics of health and wellness. He is regularly featured in the national press and has written as part of a national campaign to get men over forty into fitness.

Alex is passionate about spreading the message that there is no need to take extreme measures to look and feel our best, and that by making small, consistent improvements to our habits, we can live happier, healthier and more fulfilled lives.

⊕ www.pathtopeakcondition.com

🐦 @AlexPedleyPT

𝐟 www.facebook.com/alexpedleyacademy

📷 @AlexPedleyPT

Printed in Great Britain
by Amazon